**RE-SHAPE
YOUR BODY
RE-VITALIZE
YOUR LIFE**

RE·SHAPE

YOUR

BODY·

RE·VITALIZE

YOUR

LIFE

By Jennifer Yoels

PRENTICE-HALL, INC.
Englewood Cliffs,
New Jersey

This book is dedicated to the spirit
of Dr. Bess M. Mensendieck,
scientist, innovator, humanist.

Re-Shape Your Body, Re-Vitalize Your Life
By Jennifer Yoels
Copyright © 1972 by Jennifer Yoels and Dr. L. Larry Leonard
Photographs Copyright © 1972 by Silano
Drawings Copyright © 1972 by Lou Behan
Copyright under International and Pan American
Copyright Conventions
All rights reserved. No part of this book may be
reproduced in any form or by any means, except
for the inclusion of brief quotations in a review,
without permission in writing from the publisher.
ISBN 0-13-773663-0
Library of Congress Catalog Card Number: 73-166044
Printed in the United States of America *T*
Prentice-Hall International, Inc., London
Prentice-Hall of Australia, Pty. Ltd., North Sydney
Prentice-Hall of Canada, Ltd., Toronto
Prentice-Hall of India Private Ltd., New Delhi
Prentice-Hall of Japan, Inc., Tokyo

Third Printing..........November, 1972

It is many years since I first met the late Dr. Bess Mensendieck, and I am still astonished that her superb system of exercises, on which this book is based, is not more widely known in the United States.

I say "astonished" because we Americans pride ourselves on recognizing and adopting the best techniques in all fields. The Mensendieck System, a truly scientific approach to body mechanics and muscle function, is renowned and widely practiced throughout Europe, especially in the Scandinavian countries. Yet it has remained confined to a relatively small audience here. The reason is undoubtedly that it has not received the publicity it so richly deserves. This book should go far in remedying that situation.

My respect for Dr. Mensendieck is based on her accurate knowledge of muscle anatomy and pathology, and on how she used that knowledge to help those with physical disabilities. My respect for Jennifer Yoels is no less

concrete. I myself had a posture problem and did the Mensendieck exercises under the supervision of Miss Yoels. The result, I am happy to say, was that the pain I had in the sacroiliac region entirely disappeared, and I was able to give up the orthopedic belt I had worn for fifteen years.

This heartening experience does not mean that the exercises in this book are a cure-all, but this I do know: Many of my own patients, following my advice, went to Miss Yoels and were greatly benefitted.

Of course, you do not have to have a pathological condition to benefit from these exercises. If anything can firm, shape, and slenderize your body and also increase your vitality, it is the correct application of the laws of body mechanics and muscle function.

This is what this book is all about.

Leo Mayer, M.D.
Chief Emeritus for Orthopedics
The Hospital for Joint Diseases
New York

5

ACKNOWLEDGMENTS ✌ CREDITS

The author is grateful for the help and encouragement of Nan Lurie, Lillian Port, Alben Philips, Cecile Grossman, and the late Sidney Reinstein.

Photographs by Silano

Models: Pamela Hale
             Con Roche
             Rocci Genova
             Harry Acton Striebel

Drawings by Lou Behan

Contents

FOREWORD   5

LIST OF ILLUSTRATIONS   11

PART I: THE SCIENCE OF EXERCISING   15

   CHAPTER 1: *What Only You Can Do for You*   17

   CHAPTER 2: *Science and the Renaissance of the Body*   35

                              ✋

PART II: MAKING YOUR DAILY MOVEMENTS COUNT   41

   CHAPTER 3: *How to Use Science in Your Exercising*   43

   CHAPTER 4: *The Art and Exercise of Sitting*   55

   CHAPTER 5: *Your Standing Counts*   63

   CHAPTER 6: *You Can "Walk on Air"*   71

   CHAPTER 7: *The Arm Uses That Shape You*   77

   CHAPTER 8: *Bending Movements*   83

                              ✋

PART III: PROGRAM OF HOME EXERCISING   89

   CHAPTER 9: *How to Exercise*   91

   CHAPTER 10: *Instructions for Fourteen Basic Exercise
                  Schemes*   97

LIST OF ILLUSTRATIONS

ILLUSTRATION   PAGE

THE BODY

1   Questionnaire on Your Body
       Movements   20–27
2   The mirror perspective of your
       body   44
3   The body's skeletal framework,
       front view   47
4   The body's skeletal framework,
       back view   47
5   Some of the body muscles   48
6   The inner-margin ball
       of the foot   49
7   The long abdominal muscle   51

SITTING

8W   A slouched sitting position   56
9W   An extremely abusive sitting
         position   56
10W   Sitting cross-legged and
         tilted   57
11R   A correct sitting position   58
12R   Sitting correctly in a chair
         that has high arms   58
13W   Skeletal view of sitting
         *in*correctly   60
14R   Skeletal view of sitting
         correctly   60
15W   Sitting down *in*correctly   61
16R   Sitting down correctly   61

ILLUSTRATION   PAGE

STANDING

17W   Standing with one arm
         akimbo   65
18W   The coy forward slump   66
19W   Standing with arms crossed   66
20W   An out-of-balance step
         position   66
21W   The slouched stance   66
22R   A correctly balanced standing
         position   67
23R   A correctly balanced stance, with
         feet in step-position   68

WALKING

24W   A reckless walk   72
25R   The well-balanced walk   72
26W   A destructive way
         of jogging   73
27R   The beneficial jog   73

CARRYING

28W   An imbalanced carrying
         of a tray   78
29R   The balanced and easy way
         to carry a tray   78
30W   Straining to carry a
         camera case   79
31R   Carrying a camera case
         comfortably   79

11

ILLUSTRATION		PAGE
32W	Clutching a handbag	80
33R	Carrying a handbag correctly	80

REACHING

34W	Straining to reach	81
35R	Reaching easily	81

LIFTING

36W	A difficult and destructive way to lift an object	84
37R	Correct and comfortable lifting	84

STOOPING AND CROUCHING

38W	Stooping incorrectly	85
39R	Correct stooping	85
40W	Crouching incorrectly	86
41R	Crouching correctly and effectively	86

EXERCISING

42	The erect pelvis, showing the sitting bones in contact with a chair seat	99
43	Three positions of the pelvis	100
44	The inner-margin ball of the foot	100
45	The balanced sitting position for exercising	101
46	Correct parallel feet; *in*correct toe-out	101
47W	Skeletal view of sitting incorrectly	102
48R	Skeletal view of sitting correctly	102
49	The Median Plane	103
50	The Frontal Plane	104

ILLUSTRATION		PAGE
51	The balanced standing position for exercising	104
52	Buttock muscle, tactual aid	105
53W	The median plane in the incorrect standing position	106
54R	The median plane in the correct standing position	106
55W	Side-view of an incorrect standing position	107
56R	Side-view of the correct standing position showing the frontal plane	107
57	Rhythmic breathing, tactual aid	109
58–60	The rhomboideus arm movement	110–111
61	The rhomboideus muscle of the back, relaxed	111
62	The rhomboideus muscle of the back, contracted	111
63	Rhomboideus movement, standing	112
64	The pelvic rock, sitting	113
65	The pelvic rock forward, standing	114
66	The pelvic rock back, standing	115
67	The round forward trunk bend	116
68	Using the long back muscles to raise the trunk	117
69	The side trunk bend	117
70	The breast muscle, tactual aid	119
71	The breast muscle exercise, sitting	120
72	The breast muscle exercise, standing	121
73	Neck bend, forward	122
74	Toes raised	124
75	Heels raised	125
76	The squat	126
77	The stiff-legged walk	127

RE-SHAPE
YOUR BODY
RE-VITALIZE
YOUR LIFE

Part I

The Science
of
Exercising

CHAPTER 1

What Only You Can Do for You

This book is about the human body—the way it works, the way it should look, the way it should make you feel. It presents a concept that goes back to ancient Greece, about which most of us today are unaware.

When the average person becomes interested in his physical condition and appearance, he thinks almost exclusively about losing weight or building muscle. Yet the movements we make in our daily activities, from the moment we get out of bed in the morning until we go to sleep at night, contribute more to the condition of our bodies, for good or for bad, than the diet plans and exercises that so many people try.

This book will show you how to use your body in its common, everyday motions to achieve its maximum physical condition and vitality and to develop all of its beauty.

It should be emphasized at the outset that three major aspects of the body are inseparable: its health, vigor, and form. You may seek to improve only one, but in achieving that *scientifically* you will also improve the others. This is an inexorable law of scientifically conditioning the body. The well-shaped woman who carries herself gracefully and has plenty of vitality is also free from unnatural body aches, just as the well-built man who is strong and vigorous is free from painful aches and strains.

But the man with an aching back is likely to have an abdominal bulge, too—perhaps even a fully developed "pot belly"; the woman with swollen or weak feet is usually also afflicted with unattractive saber-shaped calves or heavy, flabby thighs; the woman who has shoulder pains almost certainly also has unnaturally sagging breasts, and the man who experiences shortness of breath from even slight activity probably has a narrowed chest and rounded shoulders.

Of course, each of us is born with a particular skeletal frame which determines the basic shape of our body, but our muscles and joints have a far more significant effect on how we look. This concept will be discussed in a later chapter.

We hear a great deal about physical fitness today, and certainly we all wish to be physically fit. But "physical fitness" makes us think of exercises, and many of us feel guilty if we do not join a gym or exercise regularly at home. Most people do not realize that they are actually exercising all day long—that the movements they make, the postures they assume, the way they stretch, bend, and reach as they work, play, and relax, are *exercises* that are shaping and conditioning their bodies, making them slender and lithe, or heavy, awkward, and often afflicted with painful strains.

The health and shape of the body are governed by a fundamental principle enunciated by Hippocrates, who is usually referred to as the father of medicine: "That which is used develops, that which is not used wastes away." This principle has been consistently reaffirmed by modern science, hence the concern that modern, sedentary living allows a deterioration of the body.

The human body is designed to move, and it is therefore equipped with an intricate musculature to perform the functions required for movement. Move and you activate the muscles.

Obviously no one can be constantly "on the move," yet it is not so obvious that when you simply sit or stand, you are also activating muscles.

It is essential, however, that you activate the correct muscles, those intended for specific functions. If you use the wrong muscles in walking, for example, those muscles eventually become strained, causing body distortions or pain, and often both. In addition, the muscles designed for walking are left unused, which weakens them and contributes further to body distortions and pain. This principle applies to all parts of the body.

But nature has been kind to us. We have been imbued with great powers to build and regenerate. Children can learn early to maintain the beauty and health of their body; young men and women can reshape and rebuild; older people can improve their appearance and revitalize their lives.

Scientific evidence of these powers led Dr. Bess M. Mensendieck to write *:

"You can now, in a sense, become a sculptor of your body, helping to shape its limbs and torso almost as though you were working with clay or marble. . . .

"This can be done because the outlines of the body depend upon the muscles which clothe the framework of bone. A heavy ankle, a bulging abdomen, a double chin—all of these reflect a poor condition of the muscles involved. Therefore, improve the con-

*Bess M. Mensendieck, M.D., *Look Better, Feel Better* (New York: Harper & Row, Inc., 1954), p. 3-4.

18

dition of the muscles and the outline of the body becomes slender, the limbs taper gently, the waistline and chest become better proportioned. . . .

"With this, you will be adding vitality and strength to the body, thereby guarding it against aches and pain that may result from inadequately developed muscles. And you will also be protecting it against certain weaknesses of advancing age. For the means you use to sculpture the body are also the means to preserve its vitality throughout life."

And all of this can be done with *little* exertion. Science has revealed the precise function of each of our muscles and the particular movements that activate them. Later in this chapter I will discuss how the customary exercise plans, which usually involve vigorous activity, sweating, and straining, frequently do the body more harm than good. The techniques presented here, based on the system Dr. Mensendieck developed, require a minimum of physical effort and a minimum of time.

EVALUATING THE CONDITION OF YOUR BODY

Whether you want primarily to improve your appearance or to eliminate aches, you have to ask yourself what form your body now takes when you stand, when you walk, and when you sit. Few people really know. The only way to begin knowing is to confront yourself without clothes before a full-length mirror. An even better method is to use two mirrors so arranged that you can get a full front and back view, but one mirror will do for now. Place a chair in front of the mirror. Now step back some distance and focus your attention on your image in the mirror. Continue watching yourself in the mirror as you slowly walk toward it and sit down on the chair as you normally would. You have just seen the form your body takes as it moves through these common activities.

But you must also know your other habitual body movements and determine whether or not you are activating the correct muscles, for the "quality" of your movements is even more important than "quantity" in the shaping and conditioning of your body.

You can evaluate the quality of your movements—that is, whether they are scientifically "right" and therefore beneficial to the body, or scientifically "wrong" and therefore destructive to the body—by taking an inventory of your body-movement habits. A questionnaire is given in Illustration 1. There you will find sixteen portrayals of the way you might be using your body in the course of a day's activities. Some movements portrayed are "right" and others are "wrong." Consider each illustration and decide whether or not it depicts your usual body movement. Then answer the question with a "yes" or a "no." After you have completed the questionnaire, you can compare your answers with those given on page 28, and evaluate your present body-movement habits.

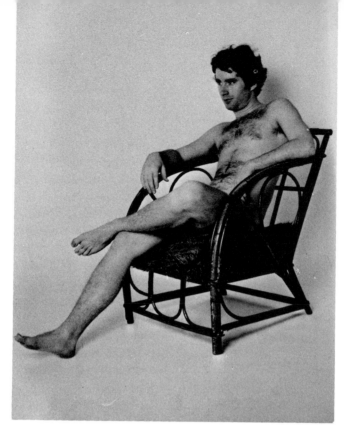

A. ( ) Yes ( ) No

Illustration 1. Questionnaire on Your Body Movements: Is this the way you move?

B. ( ) Yes ( ) No

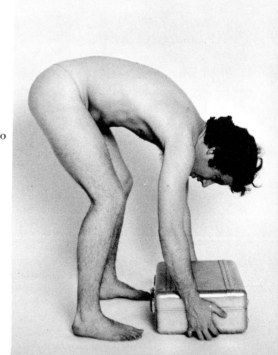

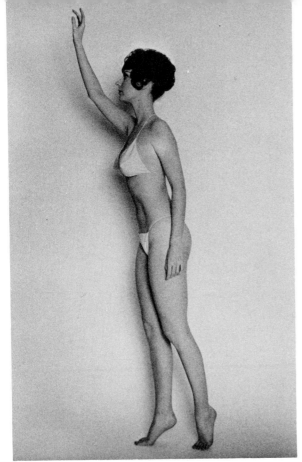

C.   ( ) Yes   ( ) No

D.   ( ) Yes   ( ) No

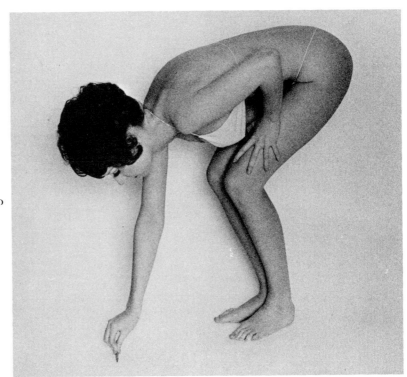

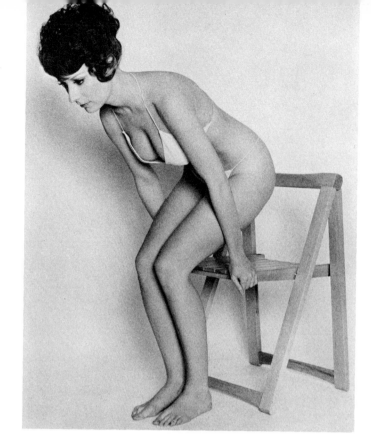

E.   ( ) Yes ( ) No

F.   ( ) Yes ( ) No

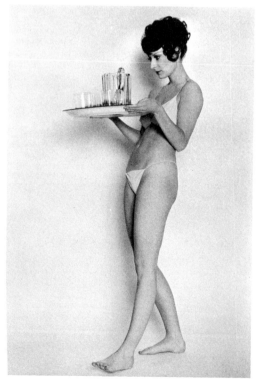

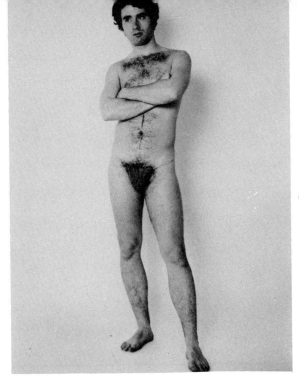

G. ( ) Yes ( ) No

H. ( ) Yes ( ) No

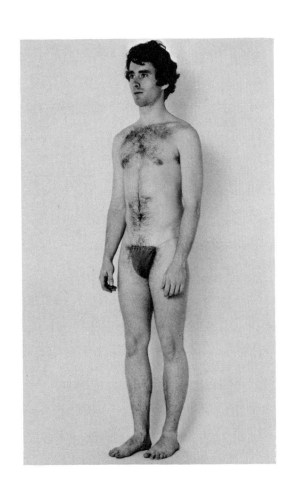

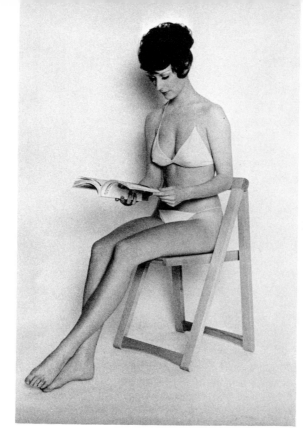

I. ( ) Yes ( ) No

J. ( ) Yes ( ) No

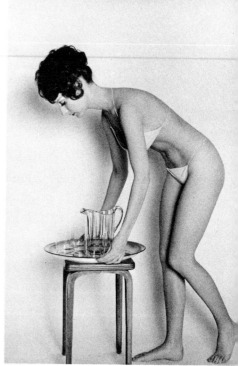

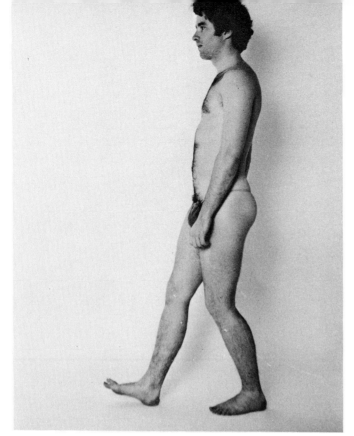

K. ( ) Yes ( ) No

L. ( ) Yes ( ) No

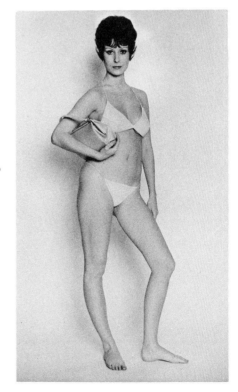

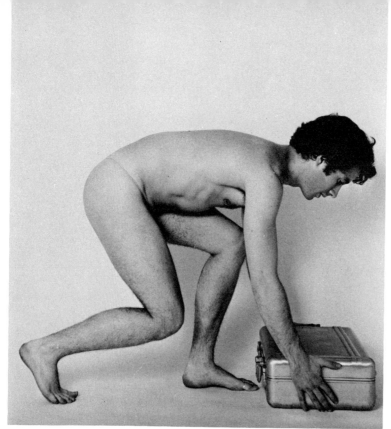

M. ( ) Yes ( ) No

N. ( ) Yes ( ) No

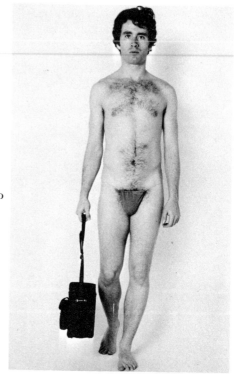

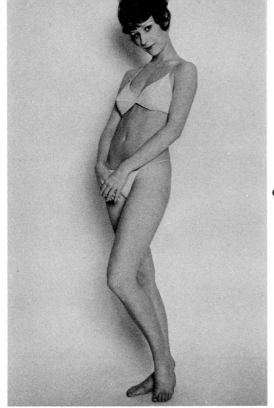

O.　( ) Yes　( ) No

P.　( ) Yes　( ) No

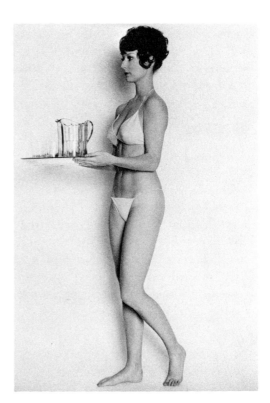

The correct answers:

A—No	E—No	I—Yes	M—Yes
B—No	F—No	J—Yes	N—Yes
C—Yes	G—No	K—No	O—No
D—No	H—Yes	L—No	P—Yes

A full explanation of why a movement is "right" or "wrong" is given in the chapters that follow. Whatever your movements, however, they are a product of habit, and your incorrect habits can be replaced with correct habits by redisciplining your body. This is not really difficult to do, but it is a challenge to persevere in doing necessary exercise schemes provided in the last part of this book. However, it is only through these exercise schemes that you can achieve the discipline necessary to acquire new habits.

Some movements and postures become habits because they are fashionable or have come to be accepted as graceful, seductive, or chic for women; casual, debonair, or virile for men. But they may also be physically destructive. Toeing-out one foot so that the feet form an L-shape befits a ballerina for certain moments on stage, but why that pose when waiting for an elevator, or socializing at a party? As a habit it is actually harmful to the shape and condition of the body. Women's hip-swinging and the recently fashionable rounded shoulders and withdrawn bosom are also destructive to the body, just as the common male stance of arms folded and one foot forward, with the body's weight forced onto the back leg, takes its toll on the physique.

In addition, modern living fosters the tendency to avoid body movement. We've moved to the cities, we sit for long hours at desks, relax in soft easy chairs, travel in cars even for short distances, use carts on the golf course. The body, meant for movement, suffers. Weekend skiing, swimming, football, tennis, even daily jogging are not enough to keep us in good condition. In fact, these activities can be damaging, because few people know how to engage in them with the correct use of their bodies.

This situation is compounded by our home and office furnishings. Although they are intended to be restful and comfortable, as well as attractive, they often disfigure and debilitate our bodies. The dimensions of furnishings actually should be determined by the body, which means by the size of the significant "body masses": the legs below the knee, the legs above the knee to the pelvis, and the arms from shoulder to elbow. Unless these dimensions are taken into account the body is strained. Even a child at the dinner table is endangered if the height of his chair prevents him from resting his feet on the floor or some other flat surface. The business executive whose well-upholstered swivel chair is too deep (the length of the chair seat being longer than his thigh) usually tilts his lower back so he can rest his upper back or shoulders against the back of the chair. This is simply inviting a bulging abdomen and the aches of a weakened lower back. The housewife who works at a kitchen surface that is too high, or the secretary whose chair is too low for her desk, pushes her shoulders out of line, rounding them, sinking the chest, and drooping the breasts.

Wherever we go, no matter how attractive the furnishings, we are in trouble if we cannot sit and stand in a position that enables us to hold the pelvis erect as the solid foundation of the spine and to maintain a level shoulder line. The problem poses practical difficulties, because obviously we cannot carry specially made furniture around with us. But by learning how to sit, stand, and move correctly, we can accommodate ourselves to furnishings and minimize their dangers to our bodies.

There are many other reasons why we move incorrectly. Just as our emotional responses are formed by our early environment, so are our voluntary physical responses, and unless we are taught and trained differently, we tend to imitate our parents' movements and postures. We understand how important it is that healthy emotional responses are developed from birth, but most of us are unaware of the importance of being trained to use the body correctly.

In primeval cultures, the individual's way of life required him to be physically alert and aware. To move slowly and awkwardly was to endanger his life, and so the environment imposed the need to move functionally right from birth. Today, however, efficient movement is unnecessary in everyday life; nimble thinking is what

keeps us alive. We drag our bodies from chair to sofa, from elevator to taxi. We use our bodies less than earlier civilizations required, but far more important, *we do not use the proper muscles for the movements we do make.*

Instead of using the trunk-bender muscles when we bend over, we give in to gravity and *fall* forward. We slump into soft, low chairs which prevent our spines from holding us up as they should. Then to keep in condition, we rush out to the ski slopes, or the pool, or the tennis courts, or the playing field; or we begin each day by "exercising," which may include lying on the floor and violently thrusting our legs into the air, then standing up and thrashing our arms about and twisting our trunks as vigorously as we can. And after thoroughly wearing ourselves out, we slump back into our chairs.

Many of us have taken to simply walking and jogging for our exercise, but unless correctly performed, even walking and jogging will only increase strain and create body faults.

Another reason that body faults are so common is that our culture places undue emphasis on precocity. Parents anxiously await their baby's first step, indeed his first voluntary movement. Baby is no sooner out of the womb than the anxious parents are wondering how soon it will be before he is able to raise his head, and as soon as he does, they express their joy and approval.

The infant soon becomes conscious

29

of the advantages of being precocious. Love and attention are showered upon him whenever there is a sign of accelerated growth. When he happens to sit up for the first time, the family's delighted approval must make such an impression on him that he tries to repeat the feat no matter how great the strain. The same kind of effort may explain the mystery of scoliosis (curvature of the spine), which, for no apparent reason, seems to develop suddenly in many thirteen-year-olds, at a time of rapid growth acceleration.

Another likely cause of poor posture and such body faults as bowlegs and knock-knees is the fact that the playpen, although freeing the parent, imprisons the child and prevents him from fully experiencing the crawling stage that prepares his muscles for walking.

The growing boy who shows an interest in his physique is especially unfortunate. He is told that weight lifting and push-ups will improve his appearance and build his strength, but instead of acquiring a well-shaped body with evenly developed muscles, his upper arms and chest muscles become grotesquely overdeveloped, making it difficult for him to raise his arms over his head and forcing him to move in an awkward, ape-like manner. The important muscles of the body—those of the pelvis—are completely neglected. This is one cause of painful back conditions suffered by "body builders" and athletes.

The ancient Greeks knew the laws of body mechanics and muscle function, and they trained their elite youth in them. If we study the sculpture of the Kouroi, the Greek youths, it is obvious that only "functional" use of the body could have produced this perfect form. The Kouros body is symmetrical, relaxed, beautifully shaped, with even muscle development throughout. Strain is absent, and the body has a graceful and dynamic quality. The knowledge of how to achieve that form was revived in the twentieth century by Dr. Bess M. Mensendieck, who devoted herself to the scientific study of body forms and movement patterns. In so doing she rediscovered the laws of muscle function and body mechanics, and devised a rational system for their application to daily living. This application of the scientifically correct uses of the body is called "functional movement," as it is based on using the muscles to perform the functions for which they are intended. Our culture, however, provides us with little incentive to move functionally. Therefore, it is necessary for us to impose it upon ourselves if we wish to avoid the aches and pains and ugliness that result from ignorance of the laws of muscle function and body mechanics.

There are other positive aspects to functional movement besides the elimination of body faults and strain. Functional movement is also joyful, pleasurable movement that adds a new dimension to living.

THE EXERCISES THAT DESPOIL

Exercise is in a sense unnatural, a technique devised by modern man awakening to the reality that his body, a mechanism designed for movement, isn't moving enough to sustain itself. Indeed, exercise as it is commonly done has become a substitute for natural body movements. Most of today's exercises call for knee bends and push-ups, jackknife toe touching, front bends, side bends, and so on. These exercises can be fortified with various equipment: dumbbells, pullied weights, rowing and bicycling machines. A measurement of effectiveness is often the quantity of sweating, breathlessness, and exhaustion endured. There are also devices for the passive exerciser—mechanical belts, for example, and wheels that knead, rub, and vibrate the body. Manhattan's current Classified Telephone Directory suggests that these ways of exercising are becoming part of the American way: It lists sixty-one exercising centers, "gymnasiums," and "health clubs." One "gym" advertises twenty-two facilities "to keep you happy while you keep fit," including: suspended jogging track, fully-equipped exercise room, gym with professional instructors, golf driving range, masseur and masseuse, Scandinavian cold plunge, indoor pool, Ping-Pong, billiard room, and a snack and health bar!

The strenuous exertions of the gymnasium and athletic field do stimulate the respiratory and circulatory systems; you can feel the pulsations of veins and arteries, the rapid pounding of the heart, and with each gasp you almost see the lung expansions and contractions. But such exercising and sports activities can also be harmful to the shape and condition of the body

if the movements called for are not performed in the scientifically correct way. Again, it is not the "quantity" but the "quality" of movements that counts.

In addition to the most common ways of exercising, many others have become popular. Yoga, for example, has found many followers. But its teachings clearly state that hatha-yoga is to be considered a preparation for the ultimate goal—spiritual development. Hatha-yoga is designed to stimulate the seven gland centers of the body, and this in turn is thought to arouse spiritual awareness. The *asanas* (postures) do not relate to the use of the body in our everyday activities. Are we ever required to stand on our heads, other than perhaps to contribute to the fun at a party? We still use chairs rather than the floor when sitting, and the "lotus position," which is recommended for meditation, cannot help us to sit correctly. Although meditating in the lotus position for long periods of time may indeed purify our souls, it will also eventually give us bowlegs. And yoga breathing may bring us closer to achieving "key energy," but it frequently causes a potbelly.

Then there is dance therapy, push-ups, and bicycling. But if the laws of body mechanics and muscle function are not applied, no amount of exercise can have long-term benefits for the body.

In fact, movements that do not conform to these laws are destructive and it might almost be better to stay in bed than to get up and move about in the destructive ways we do.

THE EXERCISES THAT COUNT

You can become the sculptor of your body, improving its shape as you increase its strength, and adding to its agility and vitality. Dr. Mensendieck proved this through application of the movement schemes which she devised and called "a system of functional exercises." With her system, even people afflicted with infantile paralysis were able to activate their muscles and move arms and legs again. With this system, too, Greta Garbo was able to enhance her beauty and gracefulness and help her body to sustain itself. The scientific validity of these movement schemes was commented upon by the chairman of the President's Committee on National Health, Dr. Paul B. Magnuson, when he wrote in 1954: "The knowledge of anatomy and the mechanics of the body displayed by Dr. Mensendieck in setting up her system of exercises and teaching the reasons for these exercises to her students has been extremely successful." And he added, "I can heartily endorse the exercises as having worked great good for many of my patients." *

Dr. Mensendieck's movement schemes are exercises in the same sense as practicing touch-typing. The typing exercises discipline your hands to type quickly without looking at the keyboard. When you see the letters to be copied, nerves transmit their image to your brain which, in turn, transmits

*Bess M. Mensendieck, M.D., *Look Better, Feel Better* (New York: Harper & Row, Inc., 1954), foreword.

instructions via appropriate nerves to the correct fingers—"a" to the small finger of your left hand, "p" to the small finger of your right hand, and so on. The process soon becomes automatic: You see a letter, and the correct finger strikes the correct key.

The movement schemes presented in the next chapters actually discipline the body to automatically move correctly. The act of raising an arm, for example, becomes an "automatism" that operates by activation of a small muscle at the front tip of your shoulder. That muscle is thereby exercised and strengthened, and its condition is evident in your properly squared shoulders. So, too, can you shape and strengthen other parts of your body with correct movements. These are some of the principles you will learn how to apply:

When you are standing, the weight of your body should be *centered* over your feet and slight pressure applied to the inner-margin ball of each foot. In this way you can prevent fallen arches while tightening and shaping your calves and thighs.

If when you are seated your weight is borne by the bony ridges on the lower edge of your pelvis, you strengthen the lower back and ward off aches and sacroiliac conditions. You also prevent your buttocks and thighs from spreading.

To turn your head, pivot it on the seven vertebrae forming the bony column of the neck. In this way your head is kept attractively erect, and you are warding off a double chin.

If your breasts sag, use the correct movements to activate the muscle that extends from the upper arms and encircles the breasts; as the muscle is restored, your breasts will be raised and firmed.

If your abdomen bulges, bending correctly in your daily movements by activating the long abdominal muscle will resolve the problem.

If your upper back is rounded and your shoulder blades protrude, use the movements that draw the shoulder blades toward each other and shape, slenderize, and firm your back.

In the next chapters the most frequently used incorrect movements will be contrasted with correct movements.

CHAPTER 2

Science and the Renaissance of the Body

Just as scientific knowledge is the basis for remedying impairments and diseases of the body, so must science be put to use to overcome disfigurements and weaknesses that are evidence of "sick" muscles and joints. The Mensendieck System of Functional Exercises is a carefully designed application of the science of body structure and movement.

How was this system developed?

As a young American sculptress studying in Paris toward the end of the nineteenth century, Bess Mensendieck began wondering why so many of the bodies of the models she sought to sculpture were marred by misshapen legs, a narrowed chest, or some other distortion. The question continued to concern her, and having found no satisfactory answer she enrolled in medical school.

Centuries earlier, vivisection had revealed the varying muscle formations of the body, but it was only in the nineteenth century that scientists began to identify the precise function of each muscle. One technique that was used employed electric current. The touch of an exposed wire sent a small amount of current into a nerve controlling a muscle; the nerve then activated the muscle to perform its particular function. For example, an electric current that led to the activation of a back muscle caused that muscle to draw the shoulder blades toward each other. In this way the function of each muscle was identified.

Through further study, however, Dr. Mensendieck discovered that many people—indeed most of those she observed—did not use their muscles to perform the functions for which they were intended. This observation became a challenge for Dr. Mensendieck to discover the "electric current" that nature might have provided for sustaining the human body. The nerves were transmitters of current. The brain was the transmission center. Could an individual use his mental faculties to transmit current via the nerves to activate a correct muscle rather than an incorrect one? Continued experimentation revealed that this could be done. For example, the arm is a lever, and the strongest part of any lever is where it attaches to the main part. The arm is attached to the body via the *shoulder*. Nevertheless, many people raise their arm from the hand, leaving the responsible muscle to be activated only secondarily and insufficiently. With the appropriate information, however, the mind is able to call upon the responsible muscle at the shoulder tip and activate it to draw the arm up from the shoulder.

With the identification of muscle functions for specific movements, it now became possible for a person to learn to use his body "functionally" throughout the day. Dr. Mensendieck further discovered that when scientifically incorrect habits were replaced with correct habits, such functional movements could restore the body's shape and vitality and keep it in good condition. There was no need for artificial exercises, gymnastics, and sports, except for the enjoyment derived from them.

It now became necessary to chart the system by which people could be taught to move functionally. Through forty years of research and experimentation Dr. Mensendieck developed a sequence of "movement schemes" that can enable you to activate and thereby exercise the muscle systems that are so important in determining the shape of your body, as well as your vigor and agility.

These movement schemes make two basic but modest demands upon you. First, you must know your muscles and the functions they perform. Second, you must train your body—in a sense program the computer in your brain—so that when you decide to make a movement the brain, via the nervous system, automatically activates the muscle whose function it is to perform that movement.

For convenience Dr. Mensendieck's movement schemes are called exercises, but they are really *anti-exercises.* They are exercises in the sense that you do arithmetic exercises, or, as discussed earlier, in the sense that you practice touch-typing. They are for the purpose of learning, and once you have learned them you don't need to do them any longer unless you want to acquire the extra benefits they can provide. The primary purpose of the Mensendieck exercises, then, is to teach you to habitually—that is, without conscious effort—use your body correctly.

Here is the explanation Dr. Mensendieck gives in her classic work on body movement, *The Mensendieck System of Functional Exercises:*

"Every individual, irrespective of his special occupation, goes through life performing certain series of necessary daily movements which must, perforce, be repeated innumerable times. . . .

"The fact is, that even the simplest movements required in daily life . . . will serve and foster the perfect upkeep of the body machine.

"Muscle development, acquired by the continuous correct performance of ordinary everyday movements *is retained until the end of life,* since correct muscle management is the basic factor of an habitually well-functioning body. . . .

"There is a certain series of the movement schemes which underlie many of these everyday movements. . . . These movement schemes constitute the Mensendieck system of functional exercises which afford you careful analytical study and training of muscle mechanism that operate to produce ordinary everyday movements. . . .

"In this way you can gradually build the body to that point of working perfection, which is the goal of all the striving on the part of physical educators." *

With increased leisure time in our society, a greater freedom of expression in the arts, and our generally less inhibited life style, there has developed a keener and more widespread appreciation of the human body than we have known for hundreds of years. Indeed, I would suggest that we are witnessing a renaissance of the beautiful, healthy body akin to the fifteenth-century renaissance in painting and sculpture. In that era, which turned against the repressiveness of the Middle Ages, the beauty of the human form could once again be revealed, giving to the world such unrivaled works of art as that paradigm of manhood, Michelangelo's monumental sculpture of David. And the Florentines felt free enough to emplace the David at the very portals of their city hall in the grand Palazzo Vecchio, without having to add the traditional drape or fig leaf to screen the groin. In modern society, after another long period of restriction, we now seem more willing to face ourselves unveiled and really look at our bodies in order to improve them.

We have gone a long way from the enforced shrouding of a patient's body with sheets in the physician's examining room, lest patient and doctor both suffer the year's imprisonment that the Comstock law decreed. That law led Dr. Mensendieck to establish her Institutes for Functional Exercises and her teacher training centers in Europe, particularly in the Scandinavian countries. There functional exercising continues to be the most popular form of exercise. In fact, in Germany the verb "to Mensendieck" is commonly used, and people frequently ask each other, "have you Mensendiecked today?" More than forty Mensendieck Studios are listed in the classified pages of the Copenhagen telephone directory, and in the Netherlands the Mensendieck System is a required course in all medical schools.

*Bess Mensendieck, *The Mensendieck System of Functional Exercise* (Portland, Maine: The Southworth-Anthoensen Press, 1937), p. 5.

But except for short intervals in Hollywood and New York when Dr. Mensendieck and her associate Amy Meusser provided their professional services to Ingrid Bergman, Greta Garbo, Jascha Heifetz, and other celebrities, the teaching of body improvement by certified specialists in the Mensendieck System has rarely been available in the United States. Therefore, I feel very fortunate to have been one of the few Americans trained and certified by Dr. Mensendieck and her associate and authorized to establish my own studio in New York. Yet in an age of unforeseen changes in the nature of daily activity, that good fortune has also proved to be a challenging responsibility.

Dr. Mensendieck lived to be ninety-six, but she looked much younger. Living to that age is, of course, unusual, but the average span of life does extend into the seventies, and in recent years I have found that increased longevity is one of the new factors influencing many of the people who come to my studio for instruction in functional movement. Older people seek renewal; young people seek not only to strengthen and shape their bodies, but to learn how to sustain their attractiveness and vitality throughout their lives. Here, briefly described are a few of my past students and the problems that they were able to solve by applying Dr. Mensendieck's movement schemes.

A famed pianist who was to perform at a concert the following week but was wracked with such pain in her left hand that she couldn't strike a key.

A successful high-fashion model with a visibly twisted hip line and intense back pain.

A business executive, golfer, tennis player, charmer on three continents who complained of a slight flabbiness in the groin area but subsequently revealed being concerned about his diminishing sexual potency.

An author completing a book under a deadline who suffered severe backaches he had attributed to deteriorating kidneys.

A woman in her mid-fifties whose increasingly sagging breasts were causing an estrangement in what had long been a happy sexual relationship with her husband.

A seventy-year-old man whose step was so unstable when he mounted and descended curbs that he was afraid to go out for a walk alone.

A muscular "Atlas" with tree-trunk like arms and with knotted muscles covering his expanded chest, who complained about lower-back pain.

A young mother who wanted to resume her career but was troubled by the continuing protrusion of her lower abdominal area and worried about the unsteadiness of her body movements.

And of course there have been dozens of men and women concerned solely about the effect on their appearance of a particular body fault: flabby thighs or arms, bulging abdomen, protruding hips or buttocks, sunken chest, stooped shoulders, thick ankles, bowed legs, and so on. Many of them were surprised to learn that one body fault was usually associated with another which they may not even have known they had.

Other people have been little concerned about their appearance—they've wanted only to be relieved of pain. One man came to my studio complaining of excruciating lower back pain which he said he had had for as long as he could remember. Having tried every other possible remedy without success, he had nearly given up hope.

I told him that as far as I was concerned his back pain was very easy to get rid of, but wouldn't he like to get rid of his pot belly at the same time? He said he cared nothing about his appearance, but would give anything to be free of the pain. When I showed him in the mirrors, that his pot belly and his pain had the same cause—a tilted pelvis and slumped spine—his eyes lit up with renewed hope and interest. His enthusiasm increased with each session, and in a short time he became so involved with his improved appearance that he scarcely remembered having had the pain.

In addition to eliminating pain, improving appearance, and increasing vitality, functional exercising also has a beneficial effect on sexual performance. Men who come to the studio are not seeking to remedy their sexual problems, but invariably they report

startling renewal in sexual functioning. This should come as no surprise, as the Functional Exercise Schemes renew the whole body, and this, of course, includes the entire pelvic area.

Until recently the only direct association between the Mensendieck functional exercises and sexuality had been in preparation for childbearing. Special attention was given to those exercise schemes that would help safeguard the woman from miscarriage, develop rhythms that would ease childbirth, uplift and tighten the breasts for nursing, and strengthen the abdominal and groin areas for the restoration of slender lines. The groin's importance to correct walking received particular attention.

Now, however, women are also seeking to participate more directly in sexual experiences and to sustain their sexual activity through their later years. Such changes in attitude are reflected in the particular exercises which now are of special interest to women. There is greater concern, for example, about strengthening the muscles of the inner thighs, not only to slenderize, shape, and firm the thighs but to strengthen and vitalize the entire groin area. The exercising of the buttock muscles is of greater interest, too, not only because it tightens the seat, but because it also helps assure an erect pelvis. And the Pelvic Rock Exercise, with its rhythmical movement of the pelvic area, is immediately recognized as being essentially the sexual movement. Many of these women report new fulfillment in their sexual experiences.

Yet there is no age limit for studying functional movement. Even in advanced age you can activate and recondition muscles that will increase your vitality and improve the shape of your body. The human body has enormous regenerative powers, and functional exercises do not demand strenuous exertion. On the contrary, the movements *must* be done slowly with periodic pauses and frequent rests for the relaxation of muscles. Furthermore, many of the exercises can be done while seated.

Children should also learn to use their bodies functionally. The ideal situation is for the parents to be trained in functional movement and then begin teaching it to the child as he leaves the crawling stage and is ready to stand and to walk. The next best thing is for parents and the child to study functional movement together.

Part II

Making Your Daily Movements Count

CHAPTER 3

How to Use Science in Your Exercising

It is said that Leonardo da Vinci in the black of night stole newly-buried corpses from a nearby cemetery, but if he did, it was not because Draculan spirits had taken hold of him. Leonardo was one of the first artists who sought to imbue his work with the natural forms of the body, and to do so he needed to know the human anatomy. Like the medical student, he had to see the actual and varied shapes of the muscles that gave shape to the body, and the attachment of muscles to joints that permitted body movement.

To "sculpture" your body, you, too, must know its anatomy. Fortunately, this doesn't mean that you have to examine cadavers or match the medical student's mastery of science. But you will want to understand enough so that if, for example, you see that you are developing a double chin, you will know precisely which muscles are deteriorating from misuse or neglect.

Then you will learn the function that these muscles should perform and how to use the movements and body positions that reach and activate the muscles. Finally, you will be given a program of simple, brief daily exercises that will discipline your muscles to be used correctly. The disciplining itself and the correct use of it in your everyday activities will enable you to reshape and recondition your body. The process requires some thought—some activation of the mind—but it is not difficult. And I think you will find it interesting, as well as rewarding.

THE NEW BODY PERSPECTIVE

To know your body, you will have to become accustomed to looking at it in a new perspective, *from bottom to top*, with a full view of the front and the back. This can be done best if you stand nude between two full-

43

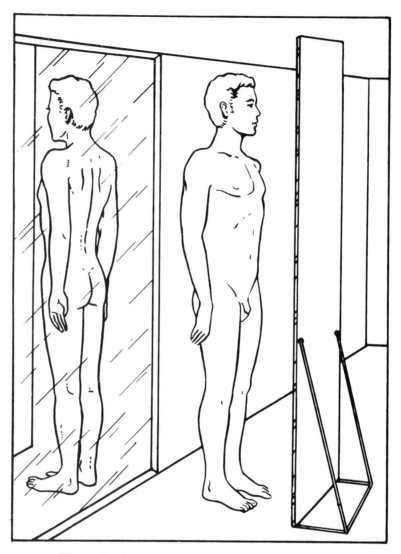

Illustration 2. The mirror perspective of your body.

length mirrors so arranged that you can see the front and back of your body completely, as in Illustration 2. If two full-sized mirrors are not immediately available, you can use one in front, although less satisfactorily. You will find it helpful if you stand between the mirrors as you read the rest of this section.

Just take your natural position of standing comfortably and relaxed. The first thing to become aware of is that the body has fourteen sections, distinguishable by the fact that each section is movable, and that their weights and shapes differ. Begin by looking at your feet and continue upward. This is what you will see (the weights indicated are based on a total of 150 pounds):

Parts of the Body	Total Pounds
2 Feet, movable at the ankles	6
2 Lower legs, movable at the knees	14
2 Upper legs, thighs, movable at the hips	30
1 Trunk or torso, movable at the hips	70
2 Upper arms, movable at the shoulder	10
2 Forearms, movable at the elbow	8
2 Hands, movable at the wrist	2
1 Head, movable at the neck	10
14	150

Now make the following observations of your body and write on a sheet of paper the location of the muscles you note.

Continue standing before your mirror, read the instructions, then make the movement *slowly,* focusing your attention on the part of the body involved.

1. Raise your toes without lifting any other part of your feet. How many toes can you raise? If you sensed a muscle when you moved the toes, a tightening or stiffening somewhere in the foot or leg, locate where you felt it (for example, outer or inner margin of the foot or the calf). Lower your toes.

2. Raise your heels and stand on the ball of each foot. Locate the muscles you sense. Lower your heels.

3. Stand on one leg. Bend the other leg at the knee and move it backward and forward. Locate any muscles you sense in the moving leg. Locate any you sense in the other leg, perhaps in the thigh or the buttocks.

4. Stand on both legs and bend your trunk slightly forward—about three inches only. Locate whatever muscles you sense. Raise your trunk.

5. Raise your arms forward and up, stopping at shoulder height; then continue to raise them until they are parallel to your head. Locate the muscles used for each phase of the movement.

6. Lower your arms sideward to just below shoulder height; then continue to lower them until they are at your sides. Locate the muscles used in each phase of the movement.

7. Bend your forearms at the elbows several times, and twist your forearms one way and then another. Locate the muscles used in each of these movements.

8. With both arms bent at the elbows, raise your hands up and down at the wrists several times. Locate the muscles used in each of these movements.

The answers you have given indicate how you are now shaping your body. They reveal whether you are forming bulges and fleshy saggings or the slender contours and definitions of strong muscles that are visible on the healthy body. If, as you raised your arm forward you sensed the muscle at the tip of the shoulder, then you were moving correctly, using the right muscle for arm raising, and thereby shaping straight, squared shoulders. If as you bent your trunk forward you sensed a tightening of the abdominal muscle, then you were moving correctly and exercising the muscles that maintain a slender abdominal contour.

Put aside for safekeeping the sheet of paper you have just used. You will find it revealing to compare your answers with the correct body movements discussed in later chapters.

SCIENTIFIC ESSENTIALS OF BODY CONDITIONING

We justly marvel at the genius of scientists and engineers who catapult a rocket into space, guide its movement in orbit, and shift it to trajectories that lead to a lunar landing—all within predictable seconds. But an even more wondrous achievement is nature's ingenious creation—man. Each of us defies the law of gravity by drawing himself up erect. And despite the continuing pulls of gravity, man is able to move upright through the space in which he lives.

The human brain, which governs man's own movement, is itself more complex than the mechanical computer that helps to guide a spaceflight. You spot a coin on the floor, you walk toward it, bend, the arm reaches, the fingers grasp the coin, and you stand up. Think of the incredible complexity all that involves: the variety of bones fitted together at joints that are themselves strapped by ligaments, the number of muscles and their accompanying networks of nerves and arteries—all used to perform that simple act. Imagine the brain drawing from its vast store of instructions the set needed to have the body respond to your request. The most minute element in that movement requires that a specific instruction from the brain be transmitted via nerve channels to activate each of the galaxy of muscles, bones, and ligaments at precisely the right time so that each part moves in correct sequence—you do not bend before you have stepped close to the coin, you do not close your hand in a grasp before your arm has reached out from your bent body.

Of course, you don't have to stop to think about each of these details as you bend to pick up a coin. When as a child you learned how to make those movements, you stored a set of instructions in your brain—you "programmed" your brain in the way computers are programmed. We all begin to store a vast variety of instructions soon after birth, and we keep adding to them throughout life. This programming of the brain results in habits.

If you habitually walk with your toes pointed outward, you've programmed those movements.

If you have round shoulders, they've been shaped by the arm movements you have programmed.

If you have disproportionately broad hips, they've been formed by leg movements you have programmed.

If your abdomen bulges, you've caused the disfigurement by the programmed movements involving your abdominal muscle and your pelvis.

Fortunately you can "re-program" your brain and substitute good habits for bad habits. The natural resiliency of your muscles will permit you to restore them, but for this to occur you must do a scientific job of re-programming by applying knowledge of the various parts of your body and their function in movement.

Your body contours are composed primarily of layers of muscles that sheath a framework of bones, the familiar skeleton as pictured in Illustrations 3 and 4. The skeletal framework fixes the basic proportions of

Illustration 3. The body's skeletal framework, front view. Note that the pelvic area is at the center of the body.

Illustration 4. The body's skeletal framework, back view.

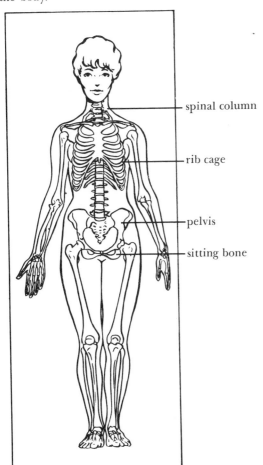

spinal column

rib cage

pelvis

sitting bone

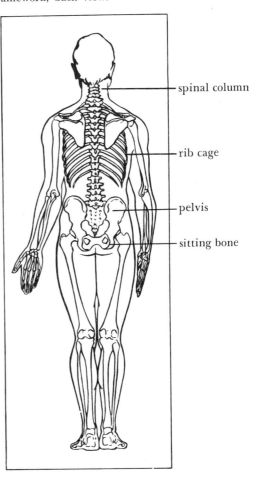

spinal column

rib cage

pelvis

sitting bone

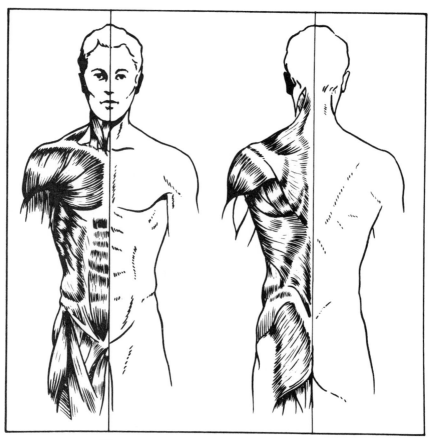

Illustration 5. Some of the body muscles.

your body—your height, the length of your arms and legs, and so forth. Within these proportions, however, you have enormous opportunity for shaping your musculature.

By the very process of standing erect, for example, you shape and condition your body. When you stand, you are holding body mass upon body mass. These parts of your body have bones that fit together at joints, which, in turn, are strapped in place by flexible muscles and other tissues (see Illustration 5). Your body masses, there-fore, are joined but movable. Muscles, however, must be constantly at work to align the body masses and hold your body erect. To do this, the muscles function in pairs, each pulling in the opposite direction to hold its part of the body in place.

You also shape and condition your body by the way you move it in the course of a day's activities. Muscles function in pairs for body movement, too, and each muscle has its assigned function. For example, the leg is bent at the knee by one muscle, it is straightened by another; the leg is moved upward by one muscle and lowered by another. The body is bent forward by muscles different from those which draw it up again. Since each muscle has a specific function to perform, it is exercised whenever a movement is made—provided that movement is made correctly.

How specific the functions of muscles are can best be seen by considering three body centers: (1) the feet and legs, (2) the pelvic area, (3) the shoulder and chest cage.

THE IMPORTANT FOUNDATION

The feet serve as the foundation for the entire body. Therefore, proper use of the feet can provide a sure foundation for erecting a well-aligned body and for activating muscles in correct movements. Should you, for example, direct your weight toward your heels, your body would be tilted. The effects of this position can be seen in several parts of the body: thickened ankles, misshaped calves, rounded shoulders, and perhaps sagging tissue under the chin. If this posture is habitual, its effects are likely to cause leg pains and an aching back.

Across the underside of your foot in back of the toes is the *ball of the foot.* To assure a firm body foundation, you should learn to activate the muscle that runs a crooked course from the bones in back of your big toe, across the ball of the foot, and up the outer side of your leg to the knee. This is the

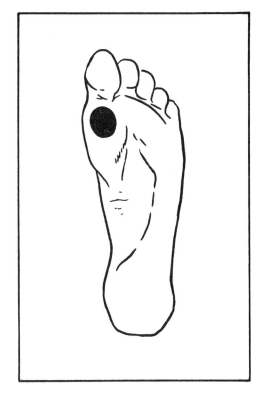

Illustration 6. The inner-margin ball of the foot.

peroneus muscle. The area of the bones in the back of the big toe is called the "inner-margin ball of the foot," and you can see its exact position in Illustration 6. From now on, when we say "ball of the foot" we mean only the *inner-margin* ball of the foot.

The ball of the foot is the focal point in assuring that you activate your foot muscle. When you direct the pressure of your body weight slightly toward the ball of the foot, your foot muscle contracts. This erects a solid foot arch. The ball of the foot is now a pillar of the foot arch, with the heel

49

serving as another pillar. With the weight of your body balanced in this way other muscles can align your body masses correctly.

Muscles on the inner and outer side of the leg now can be activated correctly to erect the leg properly from the ankle joint, and the thigh from the knee joint. This results in slender ankles, well-shaped calves and thighs, and smooth knee caps.

THE VITAL PELVIC CENTER

The pelvis is the foundation for the spinal column, which is attached to it. Therefore, the muscles that govern the position and movement of the pelvis are crucially important to the shape and health of the body. Misuse of these muscles accounts for the abdominal bulge, malformed back, heavy thighs, loose expansive seat, and awkward walking movements. The abused muscles can also contribute to backache, digestive tract difficulties, a weakened reproductive system, and slackened sexual effectiveness.

As you can see by looking back at Illustration 3, the pelvis is shaped like a basin turned on its side so that the open area faces forward; in fact, it is sometimes called the "pelvic basin." This odd-shaped structure is designed to meet the demands made upon it: It encircles the body center, and also contains the digestive and reproductive organs.

When the pelvis is erect, the pubic bone, which is the bottom of the basin, becomes a floor on which all the organs in the abdominal area rest. Incorrect standing posture causes the pelvis to tilt forward, which allows the pubic bone to move back so that it cannot support the abdominal contents. Consequently, the abdominal contents spill forward, creating a bulge or a "pot."

A slouched sitting position causes a somewhat different situation, but the results are even more damaging. In this case, the pelvis tilts back, and the spine cannot stretch to distribute your trunk weight. Therefore, the trunk weight has no way of resisting gravity, and it is pulled down. The pressure of this weight on the lower part of the trunk creates aches in the lower back as well as a spreading of the buttocks, hips, and thighs. The pressure also pushes the abdominal area outward, causing a pot belly.

Two sets of muscles dominate the functions of the pelvic center. One set, found at the seat, is composed of the buttock muscles. Most people are surprised to find they have muscles in the seat and that they can control the tightening and relaxation of these muscles. Yet it is the tightening of the buttocks that draws the pelvis erect, thereby holding the organs of the pelvic area in place. Tightened buttocks also help assure well-functioning hip joints, which are necessary for leg movements. Even when you are standing, the buttock muscles should be somewhat activated to help align the body. Your correct use of the buttock muscles for these functions will result in a smaller, tighter, more firmly rounded seat, and narrowed hips. It will also affect the contours of the abdomen. Moreover, when your buttocks hold your pelvis erect, the shape and condition of your back is safeguarded, because an erect pelvis provides your spinal column with a firm and level foundation.

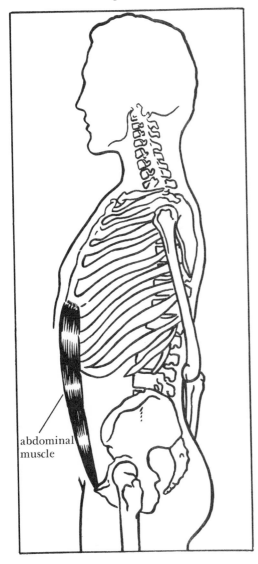

Illustration 7. The long abdominal muscle that stretches from the pubic bone to the rib cage. Notice the muscle's three parts.

abdominal muscle

The other muscle that dominates the functioning of the pelvic area is the long abdominal muscle pictured in Illustration 7. There you can see that it is a broad muscle extending from the pubic bone of the groin, to the rib cage. The abdominal muscle should function to bend the body forward as when you bend to lift an object from the floor. If you are unaccustomed to fully activating this muscle you will have to make a conscious effort to do so. The long broad abdominal muscle is made up of three sections, all of which can be reached only if the activation is begun with the lower section attached to the pubic bone, followed by the middle section, and finally by the upper section which is attached to the rib cage. Unless the long abdominal muscle is wholly activated in bending movements, it becomes weakened, and this weakening contributes to a bulging abdomen and affects the lines and health of the groin area.

The condition of these muscles governing the pelvic center further affects the whole upper part of the body.

THE SHOULDERS AND CHEST

The rib cage which is fastened to the spine and protects the heart and lungs provides the framework of the chest, but muscles determine the chest contours. One group of muscles interlace the ribs and are called *intercostals*. When you inhale, these muscles, together with the diaphragm, should be

51

activated to draw the ribs apart. This not only expands the chest, but increases the inhalation to provide the body with more oxygen. In exhalations the intercostals contract to draw the ribs together. Effective functioning of these muscles during exhalation empties the lungs entirely so that they are then capable of holding a maximum of newly inhaled air.

On inhaling, it is essential that the ribs not be drawn up; instead, the intercostals and the diaphragm should draw the ribs *apart,* thus expanding the chest *sideways.* Expanding the chest upward in breathing does not use these rib muscles, but it does contribute to a narrow chest and shortness of breath.

If you achieve a firm pelvic foundation, the spinal column becomes an erect, yet flexible, support for your entire back. Two long muscles flank the spine, and their condition affects the carriage of your body, and the strength and health of your back. These long muscles should be fully activated when you bend your trunk to the side or back.

The long back muscles are affected when you bend forward—the activated abdominal muscle *contracts* to draw your trunk forward, and as your back is being rounded, the long back muscles are *stretched.* To correctly raise your trunk erect again, however, you must *contract* the long back muscles as you draw the trunk up. If your many activities requiring the bending and raising of your body are done correctly all the muscles involved will be well exercised.

The long back muscles should also function in carrying body weight. Unfortunately, there is a rather common "sack-of-potatoes" approach to carrying the body which, in effect, dumps the weight on the legs and feet. People who use this method can be identified by the slouch of their body, bulges and protrusions in the mid-section, hips, and thighs, and frequently by misshaped legs, ankles, and feet. The long back muscles can have the strength to draw the trunk weight toward the center of the back while stretching the spinal column to draw the body up straight. In this way, the weight of the trunk is distributed as it should be. This use of the back muscles, even when sitting, exercises them and keeps them strong, flexible, and responsive. Their healthy condition becomes strikingly evident in the clear definitions of a woman's beautifully molded back and in the strong broad back of a man.

The shaping of the trunk—the back, shoulders, neckline, chest, and breastline—is partly determined by the condition of the muscles you use in arm movements. From the following descriptions, you can derive some concept of the correct way to raise and lower an arm. If you then wish to attempt the movements, make every effort to direct your thoughts to the specific muscles in your body that are mentioned. Additional instructions will be given in later chapters.

The deltoid muscles sheath the shoulder sockets and continue into the upper arms. A sector of this muscle, situated at the top of the arm in front, draws the arm forward and upward to shoulder height.

The correct method of then raising your arm from shoulder height to above your head calls another muscle into play and provides a clear demonstration of a group of muscles working together in a single movement. One set of back muscles holds your back erect so that you don't hunch over, while a rather small muscle, bearing the forbidding name of *supraspinatus,* is the one that actually draws the arm from shoulder height upward. This muscle is located on top of the shoulder toward the back, with one end attached to the shoulder socket and another to the side base of the neck. Another upper-back muscle, which extends around to the chest, draws the shoulder blades apart, making room in the shoulder socket for the upper-arm bone to rise. Thus, such a common movement as raising an arm should activate a team of muscles that shape the upper back, a shoulder, an area of the neck, a part of the chest, and strengthen the shoulder socket.

As you have seen, whether you seek to improve the chest lines or slenderize the thighs, flatten an abdominal bulge or straighten the shoulders, guard against backaches or stabbing leg pains, the scientific evidence here summarized indicates that the decisive factor is the manner in which you use your body in your normal daily activities.

CHAPTER 4

The Art and Exercise of Sitting

It may seem strange to begin a discussion of specific daily activities with the sedentary position of *sitting*. But the science of body mechanics reveals that all daily activities, including sitting down, being seated, and standing up again, involve complex movements that affect the condition and shape of the body. For example, did you know that the feet, the calves and the inner margins of the thighs, the buttocks and the hip sockets, the pelvis, the spine, and the long back muscles alongside the spine are all exercised when you simply sit down and stand up?

Even less apparent is the shaping of the body that occurs when you are seated. The position you take in an easy chair or on a couch can relax, rest, and sustain the body. But there are also sitting positions through which you may distort your body by preventing the abdominal area from being strong and flat; by obstructing

the "sitting bones" so that the pelvis cannot be held erect, thereby threatening the lower back with distortion and pain; and by permitting the spinal column to sag so that the head tilts forward and a double-chin develops.

The importance of the whole sitting activity is staggering when we realize that in any given day many people spend more time sitting than doing anything else, even sleeping. But even if your way of life is not particularly sedentary, there is considerable potential for damaging your body through as innocent an activity as sitting.

By beginning with an inventory of the various sitting positions you may take in a day, you can identify your practices, determine whether they are right or wrong, and if they are wrong, become aware of the consequences of each incorrect sitting position. By next identifying the right way to sit, you can establish your goal. Later in this chapter you will be given instructions on how to sit in a variety of chairs. In the program of exercises that concludes this book you will find a sitting position exercise to re-discipline your body.

THE SITTING HABIT

In Illustrations 8 through 12 that follow, you will see sitting positions that are typical of those we can observe every day. Each illustration bearing the letter "W" is wrong, and each bearing the letter "R" is right. In particular, look for the following:

> Is the major weight of the seated body toward the front or the back of the chair?
>
> Is the back bent or straight?
>
> Is the abdomen flat or rounded?
>
> Are the elbows resting on the arms of the chair?
>
> If so, are the shoulders raised at the tips or are they straight?

While viewing these right and wrong positions, bear in mind a cardinal axiom: Sitting correctly does not mean you must sit in a rigid "at-attention" posture. On the contrary, you should be relaxed and comfortable. Through the following discussions, you will realize that correct sitting positions are comfortable and relaxing.

ABUSIVE SITTING

How we can abuse our body in the simple act of sitting is revealed in the

56

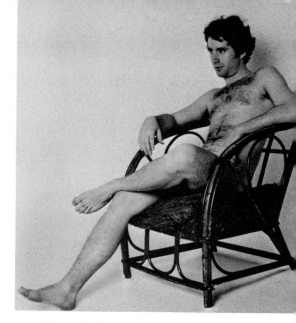

Illustration 8W. A slouched sitting position.

Illustration 9W. An extremely abusive sitting position.

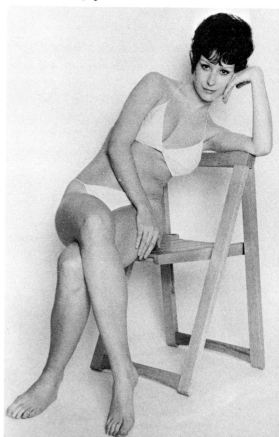

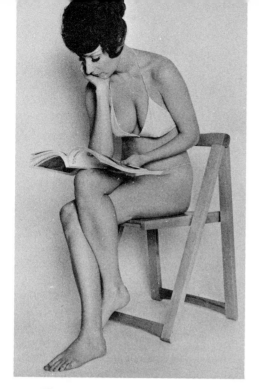

Illustration 10W. Cross-legged and tilted.

three positions of Illustrations 8W, 9W, and 10W. In all three positions, the functions of the pelvis and spine of holding the trunk erect are not only neglected but actually thwarted.

In Illustration 8W, the margin of the lower back has become the sitting base, a use for which it never was intended, and failure to erect the pelvis has forced most of the trunk weight onto the sacrum. This abuse of the body can eventually cause severe back pain, as well as disfigurement of several areas of the body.

Slumping on the edge of a chair, as in Illustration 9W, may seem relaxed, but actually this position is a very strained one. The arm resting on the top of the chair pulls the shoulders out of alignment; the chest is col-

lapsed; the pelvis is tilted back, and the body weight is thrown on to one hip. The spine is curved backward and is unable to hold up the trunk.

Crossing the legs, as in Illustration 10W, causes a curvature of the spine. Furthermore, one thigh is flattening the contour of the other, which contributes to flabbiness. You will notice, too, that the abdomen isn't controlled, the chest is caved in, and the breasts are allowed to sag. And one arm is supporting the head, as well as pressing into the thigh—a most destructive position.

The effects on the abdomen are particularly apparent in Illustrations 8W and 9W. Here the long abdominal muscle cannot keep the abdominal region from being pushed forward. The habit of sitting in these destructive positions is one of the principle causes of the abdominal bulge.

In all three positions the shoulder line also suffers because of a total neglect of correct muscle usage. In Illustration 8W, you can see that resting your arms on the arms of a chair that are too high to accommodate the body, juts the shoulders upward. The casual resting of the upper body and head on one arm, as in Illustration 9W, distorts the collar-line and neck-line.

The position which uses the thighs as a reading stand, as shown in Illustration 10W, has destructive consequences for the chest, the head and neck, the shoulders and back, and, of course, the thighs and calves.

Furthermore, the two positions in Illustrations 8W and 9W are tension

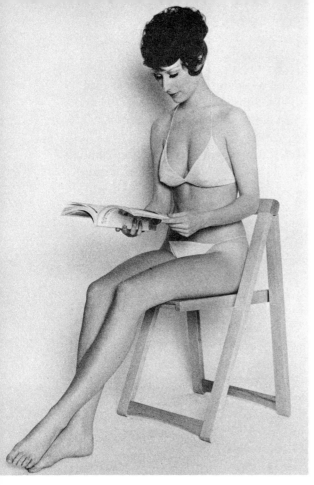

Illustration 11R. A correct sitting position.

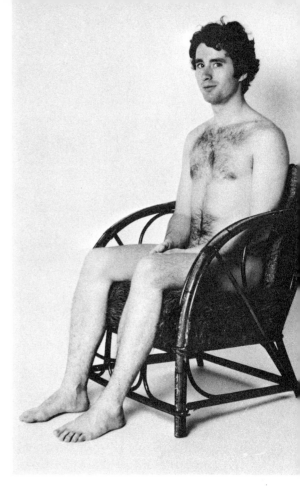

Illustration 12R. Sitting correctly in a chair that has high arms.

producing, as can be seen from the tightness of the lower legs and feet.

CORRECTING THE SITTING ABUSES

Correct sitting positions are shown in Illustrations 11R and 12R.

Notice the striking contrast between sitting incorrectly in a deep chair as shown in Illustration 8W and the correct posture in Illustration 12R. In the correct position the legs and buttocks

have pushed the trunk deep into the chair, the lower back tight against the chair back. The sitter's back is straight, the shoulders are square, the head erect, the chest high, the abdomen flat. This sitting position places the trunk on the sitting bones of the upright pelvis, and the pelvis provides a solid base from which the spine can be drawn erect by the long back muscles. And the spine, which extends to the seven vertebrae of the neck, enables the muscles at the back of the neck to

58

hold the head high. The erect pelvis also helps the abdominal muscle maintain a flattened abdomen and keep all the organs of the abdominal area in place.

The contrasts between Illustration 10W and Illustration 11R reveal that reading while sitting can be comfortable and non-destructive. The dominant feature of Illustration 11W is the step-position of the feet which enables the body to be held comfortably straight.

The back remains erect, the shoulders squared, the head high and the neck straight, the chest raised, the abdomen flattened, and the thighs tapered. This outward appearance reflects an erect pelvis with the legs placed evenly in the hip sockets, the spine placed squarely on the solid pelvic base and drawn up by the back muscles, and the muscles at the back of the neck holding the head in comfort. Moreover, the ribs can function correctly in the breathing process, assuring full inhalations and exhalations, and the abdominal muscle can function effectively.

A special alert is needed to protect you from sitting incorrectly in arm chairs. Compare Illustrations 8W and 12R. If the arms of the chair are too high, trying to rest on them distorts the body. You can see in Illustration 8W how destructive that can be. The problem is met in Illustration 12R by not using the chair arms at all. This permits the trunk, the neck, and the head to remain erect, the chest raised, and the abdomen flattened.

THE ART OF SITTING

Science provides guidelines for sitting functionally, that is, correctly, for the well-being of the body. This is not the same thing as sitting "properly" from an etiquette-book viewpoint. In fact, we hear little about sitting *correctly,* except for an occasional "Sit up!" to a child.

Although many of us live in an urban environment that demands as much as ten hours a day of sitting, we don't know how to sit correctly! Our sitting movements were learned in childhood by imitating so that dropping into a chair became a habit. The stuffed easy chairs and embracing armchairs hold us captive, yet we can offer no resistance to them, because we don't know how to sit functionally.

But now you can learn how to sit correctly. You have seen right and wrong sitting positions. The dominant lesson that emerges is that of the impact of the seated position on the pelvis. This is clearly seen in the skeletal drawings of the pelvis in Illustrations 13W and 14R. Illustration 13W shows the pelvis as it appears when the body is slouched in a chair. The pelvis is clearly out of line. Observe how this affects the leg sockets in the pelvis, and notice that not only is the back rounded, but the lower back is burdened by the weight of the trunk. Notice, too, the consequences for the abdomen. Compare these effects with Illustration 14R, which shows the erect pelvis in the correct sitting position.

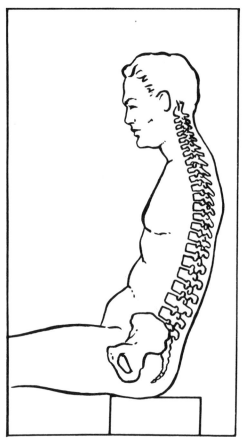

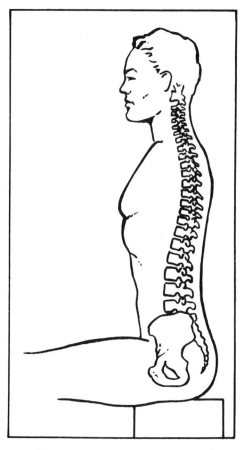

Illustration 13W. Skeletal view of sitting *in*correctly.

Illustration 14R. Skeletal view of sitting correctly.

One of the most important features of correct sitting concerns the use of what I've referred to as the sitting bones. These are two small, curved bones extending down from the lower edge of the pelvis—one bone within the center and at bottom of each buttock. You can feel these bones by pressing your fingers into the bottom of each buttock, or by pressing your buttocks firmly against a hard, flat chair. When you can feel these bones

against the chair, you know that your pelvis is erect. For that reason, they are called "sitting bones."

The movement of sitting down can also create body faults. A typical sitting method is shown in Illustration 15W: The seat of the chair is grasped, the buttocks are poked back, and then the body is dropped down. Notice how awkward this looks.

Since usually we cannot choose our furniture to fit our body exactly, we must adjust our body to the furniture. Accordingly, the objective in taking a sitting position should always be to keep the pelvis erect and the spinal column upright, as in Illustration 16R. This is how it can be done.

1. If you have a choice, select a chair most appropriate to your body proportions. When seated with your knees bent so that your calves and thighs form right angles your feet should rest firmly on the floor.

When seated in this position the depth of the seat should allow your back to reach the back of the chair. If the seat is too deep, then scatter-type pillows can be used to shorten it.

2. Sit down gracefully, in a way that will exercise the body properly and place you in the correct position. This can be accomplished by functional movements:

(a) Approach the chair and turn your back to it. (See Illustration 16R.)

(b) Place your feet in the step position, as in the photograph, with your back leg touching the front edge of the chair. Move your body weight from the forward leg to the back leg by shifting the weight from the ball of the forward foot to the ball of the back foot.

(c) You are now prepared to bend your trunk forward. This bending is accomplished by draw-

Illustration 15W. Sitting down *in*correctly.

Illustration 16R. Sitting down correctly. Getting up from a seated position should also look like this.

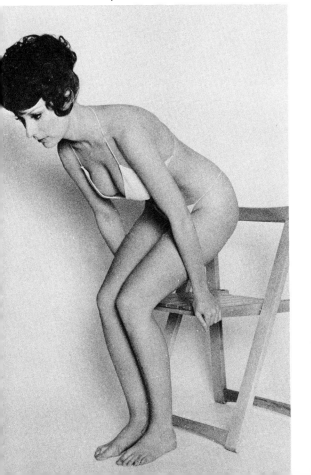

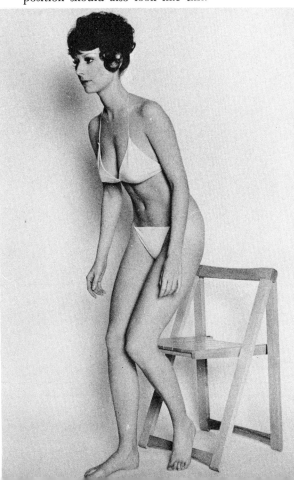

ing your abdominal muscle in and up and guiding the muscle to draw your trunk slightly forward; the forward bend should begin in back at the base of the spine. While bending your trunk forward, add the knee-bend and lower yourself into the chair.

(d) Now pull yourself back along the seat of the chair so that your lower back rests securely against the back of the chair.

(e) Beginning at the base of the spine, use your long back muscles to draw your trunk up.

In this position, with the pelvis erect, the trunk is able to rest solidly on the pelvic sitting bones. The straight pelvis and the support of the chair back keep the spine erect. The abdomen is also in place and therefore flat. The chest, shoulders, and head will be in place to safeguard the lines of the neck, the breasts, and the chest muscles, and to protect the breathing process.

This "social" sitting position may be shifted in ways that will increase your comfort and keep you from feeling rigid. Any position you take, however, should be based on the guidelines I have presented. You may even make extreme deviations, say, crossing your legs, if this brings you momentary comfort. However, *you should not remain in such positions for long*. Although sitting for long periods of time with crossed legs is destructive, you can cross your legs at the ankles without disrupting your body symmetry.

In rising from a seat, lean forward, starting at the base of your spine; at the same time move one leg back under the chair, forming a step position. When the body weight is over your forward foot, press down on the ball of that foot, and rise.

CHAPTER 5

Your Standing Counts

Even when we make as commonplace a use of our body as standing to talk with a friend or to wait for an elevator, we are either exercising our body or impairing it. It all depends on how we stand.

We can understand why this is so when we recognize all that standing involves. We are holding aloft fourteen body masses, and to hold up these body masses we must not only align them, we must also balance them. Doing this is a remarkable accomplishment, as, in addition to being of differing weights and sizes, the body masses have different shapes, and what is more, are movable. Yet they can be aligned and balanced with a symmetry approximating the ideal forms of ancient Greek sculpture.

The muscles have the major responsibility of holding us up when we stand. Like ropes stretching in opposite directions to sustain a tent on its poles, muscles are paired, and through balanced contraction—pulling evenly in opposite directions—the parts of the body are held in place. As we have seen, that is how the lower part of the legs are properly maintained in the ankle joints, making it possible for the paired muscles of the thighs to maintain the legs correctly in the knee joints, and so it continues upward, muscles actively functioning to align and balance the body masses and produce the correct standing position.

Therefore, although the body appears to be inactive when we are standing, the muscles are continuously activated. The seemingly immobile standing position, then, can be an important exercise. If we do not stand correctly, however, we are not only allowing some muscles to deteriorate from neglect, but we may be abusing other muscles by forcing them to perform functions for which they were not designed. The bowed leg, the disproportionate hip, the bulging abdomen,

63

even the sagging breasts and double chin are often partly the consequence of standing incorrectly. So also are the callous and the corn on the foot, the enfeebled groin, the pained lower back, even the slipped disc.

It is not difficult to stand correctly, nor is it uncomfortable. On the contrary, it is more comfortable than standing incorrectly, because the body is being used as it should be.

STANDING HABITS

The manner in which we stand is an acquired habit, as are all of our movements and body positions. This habit begins to form when a child, having taught himself to walk by dogged exertions of trial and error, looks about and copies the movements of those around him. Observe how like her mother a three-year-old girl stands, perhaps with her toes pointing outward as the feet form a "V," the pose so becoming to a ballerina taking her curtain call but so destructive to the body if it becomes a habit. Notice how like his father a three-year-old boy stands, the child's back curved inward only slightly now, as though trying to mirror the determined kink of the back and the modest but apparent abdominal bulge of the father who has grown to manhood resting his weight on his heels.

The copying continues into adulthood, for we are called upon to stand so often and in such a variety of circumstances that we require a repertoire of standing positions. And the "good posture" phase—that is, repetitious re-minders to an adolescent that he looks awful because of the way he is standing —usually doesn't benefit the still male-able habits. Even if a desire for "good posture" has been kindled, what is "good" and how to achieve it are too frequently unknown, and so standing postures copied from imperfect models become habits.

Some young men encounter the "at-attention" phase. Whether at boot camp or West Point, the call to "attention" brings the feet snapped together, the body pulled erect and stiff, the abdomen sucked in, the chest jutted out, the shoulders pushed high and back, the chin shoved down to hold the head slightly forward. Each such adjustment is an assault upon the physique. The military man might not suffer the full consequences as long as he continues the intensive physical activity of military life, for the laws of chance can permit sufficient muscle activation to sustain the body. But the ex-soldier whose life no longer includes the intense physical activity of the military gets little help from the laws of chance. Neglect or abuse of his musculature leads to body deteriorations not far different from that of the man who never responded to the call to "attention."

Thus our standing tends to be composed of various positions copied from imperfect models, and as a result the body is moved thoughtlessly from one habitual standing position to another.

Through knowledge of body mechanics and muscle function you can evaluate any standing position as either right or wrong. Right positions are those in which muscles and joints perform the functions for which they were designed and thus balance and align the body masses. The illustrations that follow identify specific characteristics of right and wrong postures for several widely used standing positions.

Look carefully at each set of pictures before reading the explanation of it. Try to find the right or wrong characteristics, noticing in particular:

— The position of the feet: Are they parallel, toed in, toed out?
— The distribution of the trunk weight on the legs: Is it equally divided, or is there greater weight on one leg than the other—if so, on which one?
— The part of the foot bearing the body weight: Is it the heel, the big toe area, the toes, the inner margin of the arch?
— The shape of the calves: Is the inner margin developed, or is it saber-shaped?
— The alignment of the hips: Are they level or is one hip larger than the other?
— The condition of the buttocks: Are they relaxed and soft or firm and rounded?
— The line of the abdomen: Is it flat or bulging?
— The position of the arms: Are they turned out and bent or do they hang relaxed and straight at the sides?
— The shoulder line: Is it rounded, tilted, or straight?
— The neck and head: Is the neck stretched with the head up and straight? Is the head pushing into the neck? Or is the head forward or to one side?

DESTRUCTIVE STANDING POSITIONS

Often when we think we are standing casually and relaxed, we are doing neither—we are actually distorting and straining the body. We see this in Illustrations 17W, 18W, 19W, 20W, and 21W.

Illustration 17W. Standing with one arm akimbo.

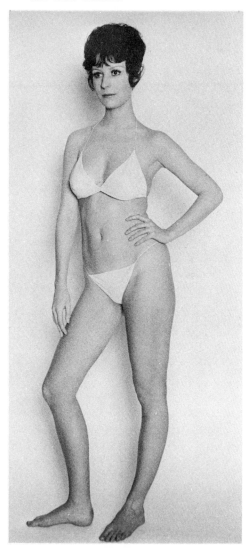

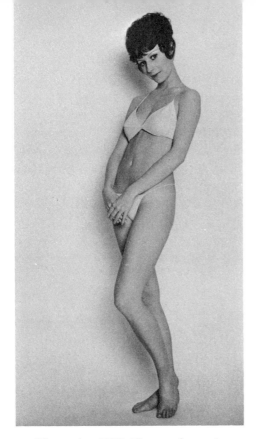

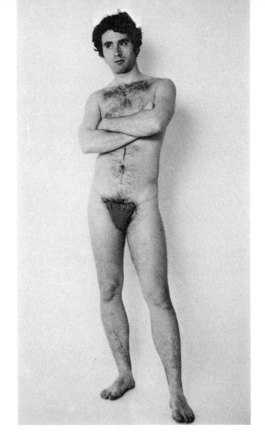

Illustration 18W. The coy forward slump.

Illustration 19W. A crossed-arms position.

Illustration 20W. An out-of-balance step position.

Illustration 21W. The slouched stance.

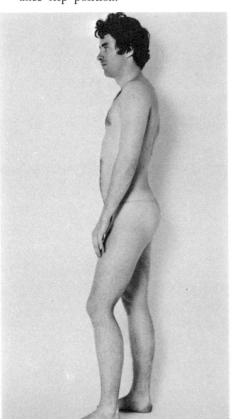

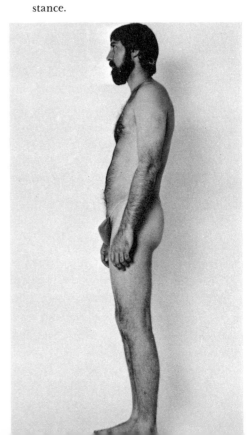

In all five positions, the body has a poor foot base; the weight of the body has been imposed upon the heels.

The foot-forward, or step, position, which could be relaxing and informal while preserving the body alignment, is so distorted in Illustrations 17W, 18W, 19W, and 20W that it imperils both the shape and the vitality of the body. In the step position, the weight of the body should be *centered* over the ball and the heel of the *forward* foot. Standing with feet together can also provide a secure foot base for the body. In Illustration 21W, however, the weight of the body is borne by the heels, rather than centered between the ball and heel of both feet.

With the body weight borne by the heels, as in Illustrations 17W, 18W, 19W, 20W, and 21W, the whole body is thrown into disarray, because the muscles are not able to guide each body mass into its proper position. In all five illustrations the pelvis is tilted forward. This produces a bulging abdomen, which, though usually linked to obesity, can also be a malaise of the underweight. The sagging spine prevents the back muscles from drawing the body up straight and tall, which in turn produces the tilted head, the rounded shoulders, and the sunken chest.

Holding an arm akimbo, as in Illustration 17W, distorts the shoulder line. Crossing the arms, as in Illustration 19W, is a way of trying to hold your body up by "leaning on yourself." And the forward slump in Illustration 18W, may look coy and appealing, but it actually distorts the entire body and encourages the development of a pot belly.

Finally, if you habitually carry your weight on your heels, your legs eventually become saber-shaped.

THE CORRECT STANDING POSITIONS

Illustrations 22R and 23R reveal relaxed and informal standing positions which are conducive to developing and maintaining a sound body.

Illustration 22R. A correctly balanced standing position.

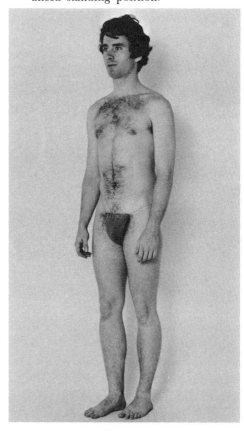

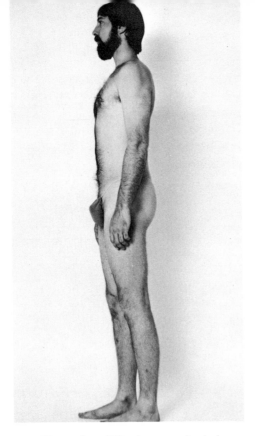

Illustration 23R. A correctly balanced stance, with feet in the step position.

The correct use of muscles and joints as shown in these illustrations aligns and balances the body. The feet are slightly parted and parallel to each other; the weight is centered between the ball and heel of the feet, slight pressure (not weight) is placed on the ball. Using pressure on the ball allows the weight to be drawn *inward* toward the middle line and *upward*, so that most of the body weight is in the trunk and is balanced over the legs. The straight legs indicate activated thigh muscles, here tightly shaped, and kneecaps drawn up. Particularly noteworthy in these illustrations are the muscles on the inner margins of the thighs that help shape the thighs and develop a taut pubic region.

The beneficial aspects of this relaxed standing position also include the flattened abdomen, with the chest high and shoulders squared. Notice, too, that the head is held up; this indicates that the spinal vertebrae in back of the neck are being held erect by neck muscles, which determine the whole chin line.

If the illustrated positions were judged wrong on the basis of appearance, some people would probably disagree with the decision. But an incorrect standing position is wrong because of what is happening within the musculature. With parts of the body out of place, the muscles are unable to sustain the body masses, and the muscle fibers deteriorate from neglect or abuse; furthermore, the imbalances and frictions of unaligned vertebrae and joints can cause sparks of pain to be flashed throughout the nervous system. Distortions and pain develop not because the body lapses momentarily into an incorrect position but because the position is taken again and again through habit. And the person who habitually takes one incorrect position invariably takes others that he may not be aware of. These destructive habits cumulatively disfigure and weaken the body, and the havoc wrought upon muscles, joints, and bones also saps the body's energy.

The positions shown in Illustrations 22R and 23R are right because they make *scientific* use of the body.

THE ART OF STANDING

Any effort to improve the way you stand involves a confrontation between your habitual standing positions and standing functionally. However, functional standing can be learned with minimal physical effort by doing an exercise called "The Balanced Standing Position" detailed in Part III. There you will discover the importance of foot placement. You will see that by centering your weight between the ball and the heel of the feet and by applying pressure onto the ball, you can draw your weight in toward the middle line and up through the crown of your head, aligning your legs properly in their ankle and knee joints. This in turn helps to position the pelvis so that it provides a secure foundation for an erect spine, which enables the back muscles to participate in distributing the trunk weight and prevent body slump.

This balanced standing exercise not only enables you to distinguish right standing from wrong, it also drives out the old standing habits and replaces them with a new habit by which the body automatically activates the appropriate muscles.

When standing correctly has become a habit, you may occasionally take a wrong standing position if it brings momentary comfort.

With your new standing habits, you will not remain very long in any of these positions or use them repeatedly.

During the time required to replace your old habits with new habits, you should try to avoid the common errors that we've discussed:

> Imposing the weight on your heels. This forces the pelvis to be thrust forward, the spine to bend back, and the head to jut forward, creating a zig-zag compensation for the imbalanced weight. The legs are also distorted when this position is used.

> Standing with one foot forward but the weight on the back heel. This, too, throws the legs, pelvis, and spine out of alignment. The thrown forward pelvis raises one hip higher than the other, which also causes one shoulder to be higher than the other. The leg bearing the greater weight becomes larger.

> Allowing the body to slump. The results are a bulging abdomen, a weakened back, rounded shoulders, caved-in chest, saber-shaped legs, and a general spreading, spongy appearance of the trunk.

> Misusing the arms while standing by placing them on the hips, akimbo, or folded across the chest. This results in an exaggeration of all the disfigurements associated with an incorrect standing position, particularly the distorting of the shoulders.

As you develop the habit of standing correctly you will see and feel the difference it makes in the condition of your body. The activation of the muscles used in standing correctly actually exercises and tightens them, thus slenderizing several parts of the body, particularly the thighs and buttocks. And this is done through the effortless exercise of standing, once correct standing is habitual. You will experience further benefits—the proper use of muscles and joints relieves the drain on the nervous system caused by the confusion of signals the nerves must transmit to use the muscles incorrectly or to activate the wrong muscles.

Thus a correct standing position brings greater relaxation and rest to the body. Finally, standing correctly means standing more attractively, for the body is properly aligned, the positions are more natural, and because you are relaxed and comfortable, you are more at ease.

CHAPTER 6

You Can "Walk on Air"

"Take long walks regularly!" This physical fitness prescription is frequently given to those seeking exercise that is not strenuous. But as we have seen, the simple acts of sitting and standing are exercises in that they activate body muscles. Walking, therefore, which requires much greater use of muscles, is obviously more intensive exercising. In fact, most of us walk sufficiently in the course of a day's usual activities to adequately exercise the muscles involved. So the prescription should be "Walk correctly throughout the day, and take long outdoor walks for the sheer enjoyment of them."

You now know enough about body movement to realize that it is not just body movement, it is not just walking, but the *way* you walk that counts. If you do not correctly use the muscles intended for walking, you are taking the chance of disfiguring and weakening your body. Walking correctly, however, can help shape and slenderize your thighs, narrow and mold your hips, tighten your buttocks, and condition your abdominal and groin areas.

THE HABITS OF WALKING

We begin to walk instinctively. Through trial and error, a child tests the uses of his muscles and joints until he succeeds in achieving a wobble and then a penguin-like walk. This kind of walking continues for about a year. Thereafter, he learns by copying the people around him until he has acquired walking habits that usually remain with him throughout life. If he is fortunate enough to have grown up in an environment where body movements are scientifically sound, then he will have good walking habits that benefit the body; otherwise he will have bad habits that are destructive to the body.

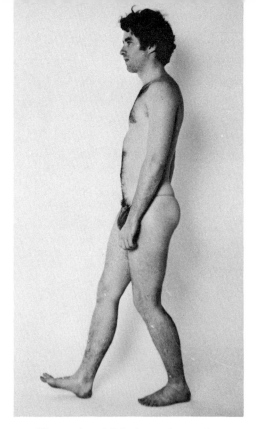

Illustration 24W. A reckless walk.

Illustration 25R. The well-balanced walk.

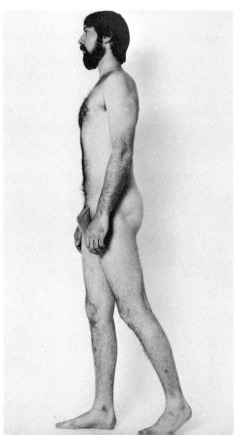

Right and wrong walking habits are portrayed in Illustrations 24W and 25R. Observe particularly:

— the position of the legs
— which part of the feet are being used to bear the body weight
— the alignment of the upper parts of the body
— the shape of the buttocks
— the shape of the abdomen
— the position of shoulders and head

Illustration 24W portrays one of a sequence of incorrect walking positions. Neither leg is in a position to allow the feet to provide a sure base for the body weight; therefore the weight is carried on the heel and unevenly balanced.

This photograph also illustrates the most common mistake made in walking: the foot is leading, which forces the body to lean back and be dragged forward. One result of this pattern is that the thigh appears spongy rather than taut.

Moreover, if the foot leads, the body's "center of gravity" for walking —the pelvic area—cannot operate to move the trunk forward in balance. Notice the flabby buttocks and protruding abdomen, both the result of failing to activate the appropriate pelvic muscles. The consequent misalignment is seen in the swayed lower back, rounded shoulders, forward-thrust head, and general slouch of the entire body.

The potential for exercising the correct walking muscles is lost in this incorrect walking.

The position in Illustration 25R is part of a sequence of movements in correct walking. In the step position, the trunk weight is balanced over the forward leg, leaving the other leg free to swing into the next step without misaligning the body. The fact that the weight is correctly carried over the forward foot can be seen in the erect alignment of the body, the flattened abdomen, tightened buttocks, straight back, head high with a broad collar line, and an elevated chest with squared shoulders. Thus the buttock, adductor, and abdominal muscles are being fully activated in this walking movement, as are the long back muscles which hold the trunk tall.

Jogging has become a popular way to exercise, but jogging can be either destructive or invigorating; it all depends upon whether or not it is done correctly. Fundamentally, the same muscles and movement schemes used in walking apply to jogging although intensified and at an accelerated pace.

The destructive jog can be seen in Illustration 26W.

From the hunched-up shoulders, the poked-out abdominals, and the hollowed back of this jogging movement it is apparent that the spine is not able to hold the body up. Jogging in this way causes the body to land heavily on the feet, which in time will affect, in particular, the ankle joints, but also the knee joints and the arches of the feet. This kind of "sack-of-potatoes" dropping of the body ignores the musculature and cannot possibly provide

Illustration 26W. A destructive way of jogging.

Illustration 27R. The beneficial jog.

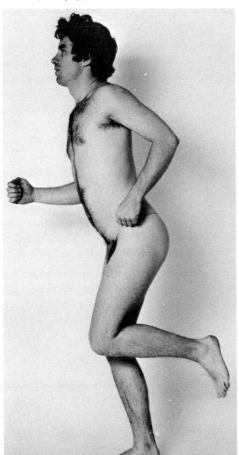

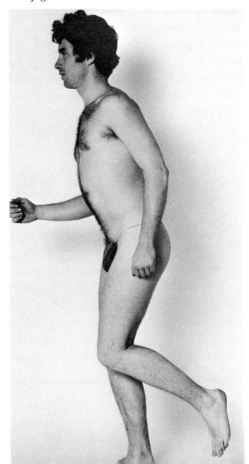

the exercise for which the effort is being made.

The benefits that can accrue from correct jogging are suggested in Illustration 27R. Here the pelvic muscles are engaged, allowing the spine to stretch, drawing the body weight upward, removing the weight from the feet. The body lands on the inner-margin ball of the foot, forcing the arch to work, creating a spring-action which travels up the center of the body to the crown of the head. The body feels light and weightless, yet practically every muscle of the body is being activated.

THE ART AND EXERCISE OF WALKING

The walking you do in the course of a normal day's activities can be of great benefit to your body. Not only does walking provide the opportunity to exercise many muscles, but by walking correctly you also ward off fatigue, since you do not draw upon muscles and nerves which were really not intended to perform in walking. Furthermore, correct walking assures a vital, attractive movement.

You can learn to walk correctly by using two movement schemes detailed in the program of exercises in Part III. Exercise Scheme 2 enables you to stand correctly, which is a necessary prelude to walking correctly.

Exercise Scheme 14 provides the discipline for correct use of your pelvis by activating the buttock muscles, the abdominal muscle, and the adductors (inner thighs).

As you apply these exercises to walking you will notice that it is not the feet that "walk you" but the pelvic area, the body's center of gravity. In a sense the pelvis can be considered a motor, with the legs and spine as principal operating parts. This "motor" directs the trunk weight toward the leg that is being swung forward. As the leg moves forward, the trunk moves forward simultaneously, which keeps the body weight evenly distributed and makes for a feeling of weightlessness. As the foot lands, pressure is applied to the inner-margin ball as the muscles governing the pelvic area swing the other leg forward. That leg then becomes the new base for the body. Then the process begins again.

Thus, in correct walking the foot does not lead. It is the pelvic center that both "carries" the trunk and swings the leg forward. Therefore, the walking movement actually originates at the base of the spine, which is the pelvis, and *ends* with the landing on your foot, then begins again.

These are your guides for walking correctly:

Make sure you are in the balanced standing position.

Press onto the ball of one foot and move the other foot, together with the trunk, forward.

When that foot lands, press onto the ball and continue the process.

74

Hold your chest high, your spine stretched, and maintain a slight tension in your buttocks, adductors, and lower abdominals.

When walking up stairs, you continue these basic movements but with some new emphasis. With each step, lift the full body weight upward and direct it toward the leg resting on the upper step. The timing of the forward shift of body weight is of crucial importance. Begin by using the abdominal muscle to draw the trunk forward from the base of the spine. Allow the lower leg to continue bearing the weight as the leg you are swinging forward begins to move to the upper step. Shift the weight forward *gradually* so that it is on the forward leg only at the time that leg is securely placed on the upper step.

Maintaining this rhythm achieves a sequential shifting of the body masses, which assures continuous correct alignment of the body. It also conserves energy and makes climbing stairs easier.

CHAPTER 7

The Arm Uses That Shape You

How you use your arms, the way you reach for or lift objects, determines the condition of a whole system of arm, shoulder, and back muscles. And the condition of these muscles is the most significant factor in determining the shape of your upper body.

To correct round shoulders, raise the chest, mold the arms, and to give vitality to arm movements, you must learn to use the proper muscles to guide arm movements. Since arm movements, like most body movements, are habitual, you can substitute correct habits for incorrect habits.

THE WRONGS AND RIGHTS OF ARM MOVEMENTS

For sets of typical arm movements are shown on the following pages, each illustrating the right and wrong ways of using the arms. They are:

(1) Carrying a tray, as portrayed in Illustrations 28W and 29R.

(2) Carrying a case, as portrayed in Illustrations 30W and 31R.

(3) Carrying a handbag, as portrayed in Illustrations 32W and 33R.

(4) Reaching, as portrayed in Illustrations 34W and 35R.

What's wrong? You can see in illustrations 28W, 30W, 32W, and 34W that the hands appear to be the predominant source of power for the arm movements. But science has shown us that the power for *arm and hand* movements should come from muscles of the upper arm, especially the muscle at the shoulder-tip, and surprisingly, perhaps, from several back muscles. The tendency to emphasize the hands in arm movements has destructive consequences for the entire body.

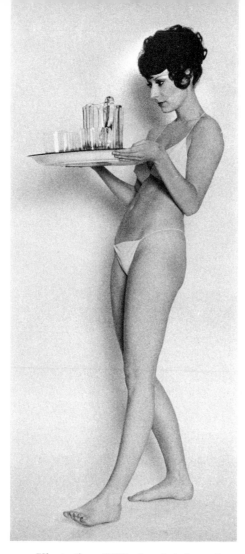

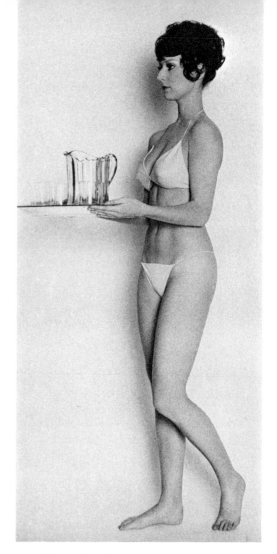

Illustration 28W. An imbalanced and very difficult way to carry a tray.

Illustration 29R. The balanced and easy way to carry a tray.

Illustration 28W shows what happens to the body. Here, not only are the hands carrying the weight of the tray, but the tray is raised to a level that makes it impossible for the arm and shoulder muscles to function as they should. And the forward thrust of the pelvis not only looks awkward, but also prevents even distribution of body weight; thus it is impossible for the whole body to participate as it should in balancing the tray.

In Illustration 29R the shoulder muscles are fulfilling their function; the pelvis and spine are erect. This assures that the body weight is evenly distributed, which enables the whole body to share the effort of carrying the tray. The result is a graceful movement performed with ease.

In the second set of movements, Illustration 30W clearly shows that the hand is doing the carrying. The entire body is pulled to one side, the weight of the camera case pulls the arm out of its place in the shoulder socket, and of course the shoulder blade is dragged along with it. The chest is also forced to tilt, and the pelvis is shoved to one side. This is the way many people carry a briefcase, a small suitcase, or any moderately heavy object. From this illustration it is easy to see why many attaché case-carrying businessmen have one shoulder lower than the other, which makes one arm seem longer than the other.

These abuses of the body can be avoided by correctly using the body as portrayed in Illustration 31R. The correct use of the arms is immediately evident by the straight shoulders, indicating that it is not the hand but the upper arm, shoulder, and back muscles that are doing the carrying. This in turn assures the correct align-

Illustration 30W. Straining to carry a camera case.

Illustration 31R. Carrying a camera case in a way that is comfortable and beneficial to the body.

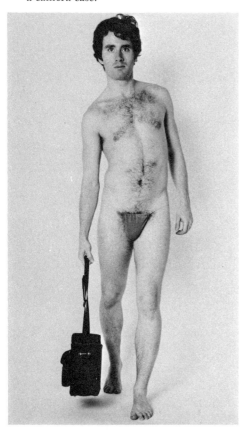

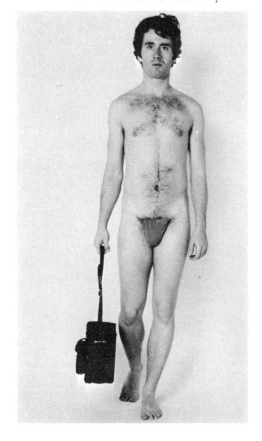

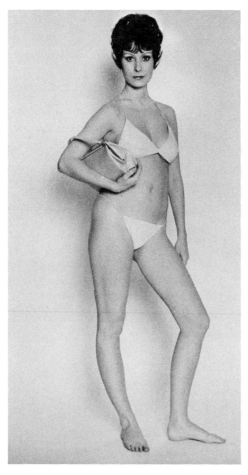

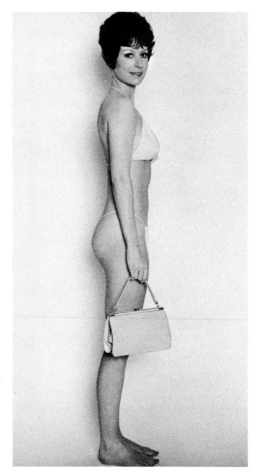

Illustration 32W. Distorting the body by clutching a handbag at the hip.

Illustration 33R. Carrying a hand-bag correctly and comfortably.

ment of the body and allows it to fully participate in the movement.

The woman carrying a purse in Illustration 32W is demonstrating a method many women frequently use—bending the arm, raising the shoulder, and resting the purse on the hip. Carrying the purse in this manner results in thrusting the hip to the side, which distorts the hipline, and forcing the body weight onto the back leg, which

produces a saber-shaped calf. This habit also causes distortions of the shoulders, flabby upper arms, and disfigurement of the bust-line.

Actually, the correct method of carrying a purse or small parcel is quite simple, as we can see in Illustration 33R. The secret lies in *carrying* and not *clutching*. This means that the arm does the carrying, and the hand merely *holds* the parcel.

80

Our fourth portrayal of a common error in arm movements involves the act of reaching above the head. Notice that in Illustration 34W, the hand is once again left to do the work. The shoulder muscles are completely ignored, even though they have the power to perform this function. Reaching also requires use of the legs and the ball of each foot—and failure to do so imposes an unnecessary strain on the body.

Compare this reaching movement with the correct one in Illustration 35R. Here we see the whole body participating—from the ball of the foot upward. The step position provides a wide base; the arm is drawn up from the shoulder socket and at the same time pressure is applied to the ball of the forward foot. This way of reaching fully utilizes all the muscles of the body and achieves maximum elasticity with a minimum of strain.

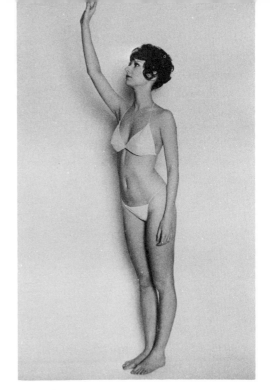

Illustration 34W. Straining to reach.

Illustration 35R. An easy reach that improves the body.

CONSTRUCTIVE ARM USES

The system of the body used for moving the arms—the muscles of the hands, arms, shoulders, back, the related bones and joints—functions correctly only as part of the whole body mechanism. This and other body systems are similar to an automobile's wheel and brake system, which has no operational capability in the functioning of the car apart from the total mechanism. In the body, furthermore, the condition of one part affects many others. A weakened ankle or a loose

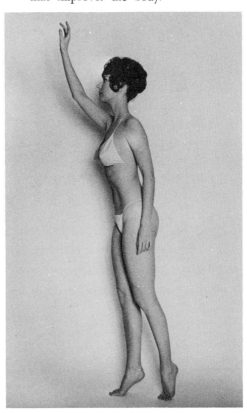

hip socket, for example, contributes to rounding the shoulders and poor functioning of the shoulder socket. Therefore the body must function well as a whole, with muscles and joints being activated and exercised from the ball of the foot to the head.

How to use your arms so that your whole body benefits can be learned through the program of exercises detailed in Part III.

Exercise Scheme 4 activates a group of muscles used in arm movements. Among these muscles are the deltoids, the rhomboideus, the trapezius, and the latissimus, which will be identified and discussed more fully with the exercises. The condition of these muscles affects the shape of the arms, shoulders, and back.

Exercise Scheme 10 reaches the muscle called the pectoralis. The use of this muscle is particularly significant in developing and shaping the chest and breasts.

Until the exercises are mastered, you will benefit from these interim guides to the use of your arms.

(1) The entire body, for the ball of the foot upward, should participate in all arm movements.

(2) The movement of the arm itself should originate at the shoulder socket.

(3) The step position should always be used, and the trunk weight should be balanced over the *forward* leg.

(4) In reaching upward, press down on the ball of the forward foot at the moment of reaching to create a spring action.

(5) In carrying an object, use a stretched rather than a bent arm, and be sure that the shoulders are level.

(6) When not in use the arms should always hang at the sides.

In all these movements try to be relaxed and comfortable, aware that when they become automatic they will provide your body with daily exercise.

CHAPTER 8

Bending Movements

The most obvious effect of bending incorrectly is the common and distressing abdominal bulge. Toe-touching has long been a popular way of attempting to combat the bulge. In this exercise the trunk is swung forward swiftly in a great stretching exertion and an attempt is made to touch the floor with the fingers.

This exercise, however, is actually counter to the scientific use of the body. The result of the movement is that it often disfigures more than it restores, harms more than it strengthens. In fact, this kind of bending actually encourages the development of a bulge, because no effort is made to use the trunk-bending muscle, which is the abdominal muscle itself. Instead, the trunk is either flung forward or it is allowed to give in to gravity and fall forward. Toe-touching exercises can also affect other parts of the body, causing saber-shaped legs, slumped shoulders, and a misshaped upper back.

There are many daily activities that require bending correctly, and all of these activities could provide the exercise you need for a shaped, slender waistline and a flat abdomen.

The most important point to learn is that all bending movements should originate at the base of the spine, with the abdominal muscle used to draw the body forward. The bend can be as slight as in a handshake or in reaching for the phone, or it can be an extended bend, as in stooping to pick something up off the floor. It is the way these bending movements are accomplished that is crucial to the condition of your body.

RIGHT AND WRONG BENDING

Illustrations 34 through 39 show

the right and wrong way to bend in the following situations:

(1) Lifting a tray, Illustrations 36W and 37R.

(2) Stooping, Illustrations 38W and 39R.

(3) Crouching, Illustrations 40W and 41R.

LIFTING A TRAY. Notice the position of the feet in Illustration 36W. Rather than placed in the step position, the feet are held together, depriving the body of a correct base. This misuse of the feet is further aggravated by having the heels bear the body weight, which distorts the alignment of the legs, pelvis, spine, and shoulders. This prevents the arms from participating with the body in carrying the tray with grace and ease.

In Illustration 37R you can see how the step position allows the lifting to be done more easily. By sustaining the body weight over the forward leg,

Illustration 36W. A difficult and destructive way to lift an object.

Illustration 37R. Correct and comfortable lifting.

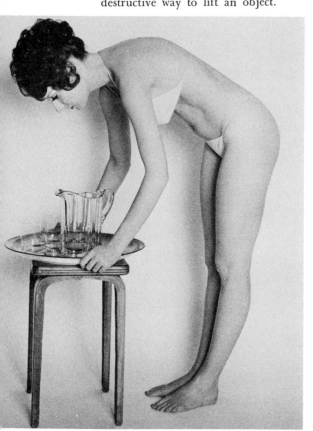

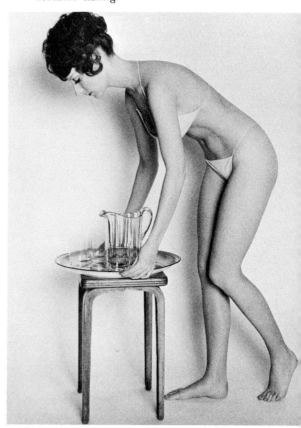

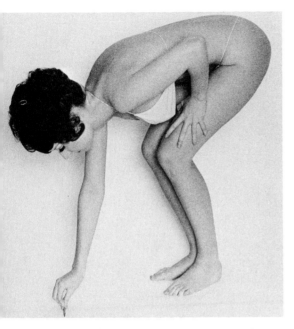

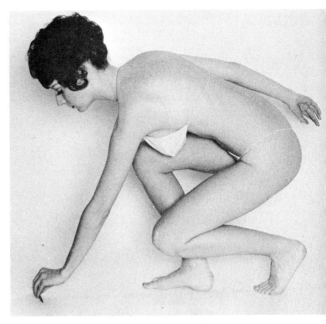

Illustration 38W. Distorting the body while attempting to stoop.

Illustration 39R. Correct stooping. Notice the gracefulness of this movement.

the entire body is balanced and can participate in the lifting. As a result, there is less strain on the body and the tray actually seems lighter.

STOOPING. Since we stoop so often in a day's activities, the misuse of the body in Illustration 38W has particular significance. Once again the foot base is faulty. Even more destructive is that the body is allowed to give in to gravity and is flung forward. One consequence is a bulging abdomen. Illustration 39R shows how to stoop correctly and easily. With the body supported by the strong foot-forward

base, the abdominal muscle is able to perform its function of drawing the trunk forward.

CROUCHING. Crouching is an extension of stooping, and when lifting is involved, the foot base is of particular importance. The strain and awkwardness evident in Illustration 40W comes from a foot base which, although wide, is not in step position. Again the body has submitted to gravity rather than using those muscles it should in lifting a heavy object. Notice the bulging abdomen and the hunched shoulders.

When the correct step position is

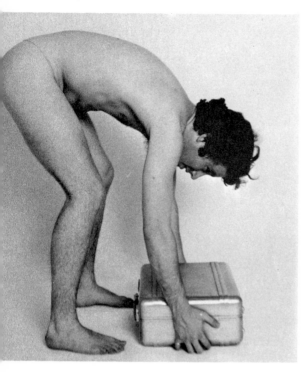

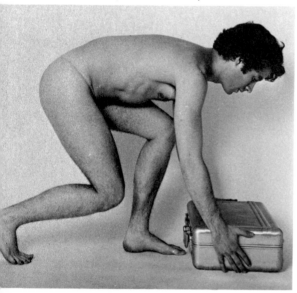

Illustration 40W. A strained and distorted way to crouch.

Illustration 41R. Crouching correctly and effectively.

used, as in Illustration 41R, the harmony of body movement is apparent. The muscles of the legs, abdomen, and back are fully activated, and the arms are used correctly. This scientific and functional use of the body in bending has the effect of making a heavy object seem light.

CORRECT BENDING GUIDES

The habits of bending correctly can be learned from the following exercises detailed in Part III:

The Round Forward Trunk Bend, Exercise Scheme 8, develops the abdominal muscle and the long back muscles. The tonic condition of these muscles safeguards the body against abdominal bulge and lower back pain.

Exercise Scheme 13, the Squat, makes leg movements strong and elastic. This exercise is especially effective in strengthening and shaping the thighs and calves and in helping to build the arch of the foot.

As these exercises create new habits, correct bending will become automatic. Meanwhile the following lines will help you safeguard your body while bending, stooping, and crouching:

1. Center yourself in front of the object while walking toward it.

2. Stop in the step position when you are near the object.

3. Tighten the buttocks and adductors and draw the lower abdomen *in and up.*

4. Press down on the ball of the forward foot and, by using the abdominal muscle, simultaneously draw the trunk forward, starting at the base of the spine.

5. Add the knee-bend so that both the trunk and legs participate in the bending action.

6. Keep the shoulders down as the arm (or arms) reach for the object.

7. Complete the action by pressing again on the ball of the forward foot as you stretch the trunk and knees up, returning to an erect position.

8. Since you are already in the step position, you can now walk forward with the object.

Part **III**

❧

Program
of Home
Exercising

CHAPTER 9

How to Exercise

In the preceding chapters it has been shown that your movements during an ordinary day's activities can actually weaken and disfigure your body. It has also been shown, however, that if done correctly, your movements will be constructive and regenerative—they will remodel your body, while restoring its vitality and agility—because you are using your body in accordance with scientific principles.

Now that you have seen the evidence and read the explanations, you should be ready for the basic exercises. With these you can discipline your body for the new ways you will use it, while at the same time giving it added opportunity for improvement.

AN EDUCATION IN MOVING THE BODY

The basic goal of the Mensendieck System of Functional Exercises now being taught at the Yoels Studio is that you learn to use your body with comfort and ease for its own betterment. You learn which muscles and joints are involved in the body's principal movements, you receive training in activating the correct muscles, and you learn how to apply your newly learned movements to daily activities. Thus one of the unique features of these exercises is that once you have made complete use of them to retrain your body, your normal activities will be your exercises throughout your waking hours. No further exercises should be necessary, except for specific purposes that will be discussed later. You may engage in jogging, bicycling, and many other physically strenuous activities (and indeed have more energy to perform them) solely for the enjoyment and added stimulation they bring. But you will also have the added advantage of applying the knowledge of your body to safeguard it against the potentially damaging effects of some exercises and sports.

Since our exercise system, then, is really a course in how to use your body correctly, this book is similar to a manual. It is an alternative to attending classes and may be the only way the course can be taken. If you strive to follow the instructions precisely, you should be able to benefit greatly from this manual.

Our exercise system enables you to identify the specific muscle to be activated in the movements of each exercise scheme. To reach a muscle you should know as much about it as you can, but as a hobbyist rather than a professional. Therefore, it is helpful to know the major muscles by name. You will find, for example, that on the inner margin of each thigh, extending from the groin to the knee, is the adductor muscle. These muscles have a specific function in standing, bending, walking, and in balancing your body. They are also important in shaping the thighs and in determining the condition of the groin area, which affects the sexual organs and processes. Several of the exercise schemes require that the adductors be activated.

To activate any muscle, however, it is not only necessary to "call" to the muscle, preferably by name, but to direct all your attention to carefully guiding the activation of the muscle in *slow* movements. *Slow* is a key word that cannot be overstressed. Unless the movement is done slowly, the

muscle being sought cannot be effectively controlled or activated—in fact, it may not be activated at all.

THE NECESSITY OF CONFRONTING YOURSELF IN MIRRORS

The whole process of identifying and activating muscles is facilitated by direct observation of body movements through the aid of mirrors. At the Yoels Studio several mirrors are used to permit observation of movements and muscles from the front, side, and rear. The rear mirror is swiveled so that by looking into the front mirror the student has a three-quarter view of his back. If you have a full-length mirror at home, you can use a spring-tensioned pole (the type used for book shelves) to sustain another mirror that can be swiveled into a position that allows the two mirrors together to provide you with a front and back view of your body. The combination of the call upon a muscle and the direct observation of your body contributes to more accurate activation and use of the muscle. At least a single full-length mirror is essential.

MINIMIZING PHYSICAL EXERTION

The movements in these exercise schemes are not only deliberate and slow, they are also mild, requiring little physical exertion. For example, as you look into the mirrors while moving your arms down in Exercise Scheme 5, you may be surprised to see muscle outlines heighten as a groove forms down the center of the back. Some movements in which the muscles are being fully activated may cause parts of the body to redden slightly, and after the first few exercises your muscles may also ache slightly until they have been toned. But there is no jumping, arm swinging, rapid trunk bending, hanging from bars, lifting or balancing of paraphernalia. The characteristics that distinguish the exercise schemes from all other exercises is exemplified by some of their names —for example, "The Balanced Sitting Position," "Rhythmic Breathing," "The Balanced Standing Position." It is control, rather than exertion, that is vital in the exercises that follow—and that control is based on knowledge.

THE INDIVISIBILITY OF SHAPE AND VITALITY

The exercise schemes are directed to the body as a whole so that it can achieve its fullest potential. Therefore you will even be doing foot movements and head movements, along with many others. The science of anatomy indicates it could be no other way, for the several limbs and sections of the body are not separate but interdependent.

Indeed, anyone seeking to remedy a bulging abdomen permanently would be striving in vain if he did not direct some of his attention to the inner-margin ball of the foot. Anyone seeking to eliminate a double chin and reduce facial wrinkles must concentrate on seven vertebrae that continue the spine into the neck, as well as on the two sitting bones that jut from the pelvis for the correct sitting position. Therefore, in this process of reshaping and reinvigorating to achieve the specific goals you had in mind initially, changes will be made throughout the body. Destructive and ungainly patterns of movement will be "unlearned" and replaced by rhythmic ones in tune with a totally harmonious body. You will learn from the exercise schemes how to stand, sit, walk, bend, and reach *functionally*—that is, how to use your body parts in conformity with the patterns nature intended. Some of these changes will be apparent quite early, others will take longer to bring about.

EXERCISING FOR SPECIFIC NEEDS

The exercise schemes can be used on a sustained basis for continuing body improvement, for special muscle needs not otherwise fulfilled, and for physical therapy. Although the course has essentially been completed when you have mastered the exercise schemes and applied them to your daily activities, you may wish to have "refresher" sessions. These will help to ward off a kind of despoliation of the body that the environment tends

93

to perpetrate with house furnishings, shoe and clothing styles, streets, stairs, cars that too often ignore the qualities that would make them beneficial to the body.

Doing selected exercise schemes daily after you have completed the course is also valuable in reaching muscles and joints that usually are not sufficiently activated in a normal day's movements. For example, the pectoralis muscle, which is vital to sustaining uplifted breasts, ordinarily is activated only minimally. Accordingly, I have included a section which identifies the five exercise schemes that I usually recommend as both refresher and supplementary exercises to daily movements.

The third reason for continuing the exercise schemes is to improve specific defects in the esthetic or physical condition of the body. While the primary goal of the System of Functional Exercises is to teach proper body movement, serious disfigurements—such as a pot belly and expansive buttocks—can be corrected by continuing to do exercise schemes specially selected for a particular body fault. These "corrective" uses of the exercise schemes should be continued after you have completed the basic course until the defect is remedied.

HOW TO BENEFIT FROM THE EXERCISES

The fourteen basic exercises detailed on the following pages should be done daily and in the order given until the correct movements become automatic. You will be guided step-by-step through all the exercises, helping assure your precision by identifying the muscles involved, describing their functions, and alerting you to the difficulties in certain movements.

These are the basic guidelines to learning the exercise movements:

1. A time should be set for doing the exercise schemes each day, preferably in the mornings. A half hour, or as close to it as your schedule permits, is reasonable.

    After two months you may find you can reduce the time, but ten minutes each day should be the minimum.

2. The fourteen exercise schemes should be done for two months in the order they are given. During the first two weeks only three exercise schemes should be done in a day.

3. Read the full text of the exercise scheme you are about to do. Then do the exercise scheme twice, consulting the book as needed. Rest for a minute and do the exercise scheme twice again without the use of the book if possible.

4. You should be unclothed while doing the exercises. Only in this way can you be in contact with your body and become aware of the muscles that need to be activated.

5. The exercises should be done between two full-length mirrors so that you can have a full front and

94

rear view of your body. If two mirrors cannot be obtained, one mirror in front should be used. The only other equipment needed is a stool or a straight armless chair with a firm, flat seat.

6. Do each exercise scheme slowly, a phase at a time, in the order given. Remember, your goals are not sweat and strain but achieving precision and complete control of the movement. Therefore, ask yourself, "What area of the body am I concerned with?" "What movement do I want to make?" "What muscle do I want to activate to make the movement?" "Am I making the movement correctly?"

7. Remember, too, that your goal is to shape your muscles by developing them. A muscle is developed by the alternating processes of contraction and release. But each of these processes must be under your control at all times, which means contraction and release must be carefully paced. Contraction should not be a kind of quick shove of the muscle, and release should not be a quick dropping of the muscle. Instead you need to be constantly aware of the specific muscle used, and you must slowly guide its contraction and then slowly guide its release.

8. Keep your eyes constantly on your mirror image. Look into the front mirror to assure the symmetry of your body—that you are not tilting forward or back or to one side or the other; that your pelvis is not poking out to one side; that one shoulder is not higher than the other. Your body must be straight, as though your straightness would match up with a plumb line from the ceiling to the floor.

Keep in mind that your body cannot accept everything at once, particularly when it has to unlearn habits that have been used for years, and when it has to reach a muscle long dormant and therefore elusive. You are guiding your body through a gradual learning process, so be patient, knowing that science is on your side.

You are about to begin a course of self-betterment that will provide an interesting experience and bring you lifetime rewards. You will probably "meet" your body for the first time—that is, know what makes it move. As you progress through the fourteen exercise schemes you will observe many changes—some obvious, others subtle —in the way you look and feel.

CHAPTER 10

Instructions for
Fourteen Basic
Exercise Schemes

You are now prepared for the fourteen basic exercise schemes. Some of these can be done in both the sitting and the standing positions.

I recommend that you do the sitting version of the exercise first until you have mastered the new movement. Thereafter, do the standing version exclusively, except under special circumstances, such as when you are tired or feel weak due to illness or other causes.

Do the exercise schemes in the order that they are given.

To learn the system as a whole, each new exercise should be learned gradually. Therefore, a week-by-week sequence is given below.

Do the exercise schemes every day —mornings if possible.

Do each exercise scheme twice, then rest, and do twice again.

First Week:
1. Exercise Scheme 1: The Balanced Sitting Position

2. Exercise Scheme 2: The Balanced Standing Position

3. Exercise Scheme 3: Rhythmic Breathing, Sitting

4. Exercise Scheme 4: The Rhomboideus, Sitting

5. Exercise Scheme 5: The Rhomboideus, Standing

Second Week:

1. Exercise Scheme 4: The Rhomboideus, Sitting

2. Exercise Scheme 5: The Rhomboideus, Standing
(The Balanced Sitting Position, the Balanced Standing Position, and Rhythmic Breathing exercises are no longer done separately, since they constitute a part of all further exercises.)

3. Exercise Scheme 6: The Pelvic Rock, Sitting

4. Exercise Scheme 7: The Pelvic Rock, Standing

Third Week:

Repeat the exercises of the previous week and add the following:

Exercise Scheme 8: The Round Forward Trunk Bend

Fourth Week:

Repeat the previous exercises and add the following:

Exercise Scheme 9: The Side Trunk Bend,

a. Sitting

b. Standing

Fifth Week:

Repeat the previous exercises and add the following:

Exercise Scheme 10: The Breast Muscle Exercise,

a. Sitting

b. Standing

Sixth Week:

Repeat the previous exercises and add the following:

Exercise Scheme 11: The Chin Line Exercises,

a. Round Forward Neck Bend

b. Side Neck Bend

Seventh Week:

Repeat the previous exercises and add the following:

Exercise Scheme 12: Foot Exercises,

a. Toe Raising, Sitting

b. Heel Raising, Sitting

c. Heel Raising, Standing

Eighth Week:

Repeat the previous exercises and add the following:

Exercise Scheme 13: The Squat

Ninth Week:

Repeat the previous exercises and add the following:

Exercise Scheme 14: The Stiff-Legged Walk,

a. Forward

b. Backward

c. Sideward

Do all the exercise schemes every day for one more month.

After that, to keep in the best possible condition, the following exercises should be done daily in the order given:

1. Exercise Scheme 4: The Rhomboideus, Sitting

2. Exercise Scheme 8: The Round Forward Trunk Bend

3. Exercise Scheme 9: The Side Trunk Bend, Standing

4. Exercise Scheme 13: The Squat

5. Exercise Scheme 14: The Stiff-Legged Walk; Forward, Backward, Sideward

To these basic five exercises, add the exercises appropriate to any particular personal problems that require your special attention. For example:

Sagging Breasts—Exercise Scheme 10: The Breast Muscle Exercise

Double Chin—Exercise Scheme 11: The Chin Line Exercises

Fallen Arches—Exercise Scheme 12: Foot Exercises

Most other problems can be corrected by doing the five basic exercises. But by this time you probably see the relationship of the exercises to particular body faults.

THE BUTTOCK MUSCLE. The buttock muscle is of special importance because its development holds the pelvis erect, therefore, it should be worked on at every possible opportunity, such as when you are waiting to cross the street, waiting on line, waiting for or riding in an elevator, and so forth. It is important to remember, however, that the buttock muscle exercising should be done only when standing still—never when sitting or moving about. Don't hesitate to do this exercise in public, as clothing hides the tension and release of the muscle.

First make sure that the foot base is established (parallel foot placement and ball pressure), then slowly tighten and release the buttocks. Repeat the contraction and release slowly and in rhythm as many times as possible. There is no limit for the development of this muscle. Work at it whenever you get a chance, and make it a lifetime habit.

BALANCED SITTING

The aim here is twofold:
First, to achieve the proper alignment of the several parts of your body in the seated position, and

Second, to train the spine to hold up the upper part of your body.

In the standing position the body is supported by the feet.

In the seated position the trunk alone need be supported. This support is given by the erect pelvis resting on the chair.

There is a particular part of the body which is the contact point between pelvis and seat. It is the lower part of the pelvis, from which jut two bones. These are appropriately called the "sitting bones." When your sitting bones are in proper contact with the seat, as in Illustration 42, you are sitting squarely on the buttocks, rather than allowing any of the weight to shift toward the thighs.

To find or to become aware of the sitting bones via tactual aid, sit toward the forward edge of a stool or a firm, flat, armless chair. The chair height

Illustration 42. The erect pelvis, showing the sitting bones in contact with a chair seat.

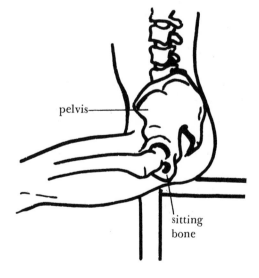

pelvis—

sitting bone

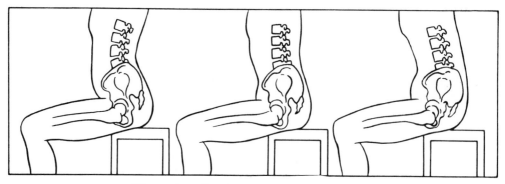

Illustration 43. Three positions of the pelvis.

should be the height of your legs, from heels to knees.

Glide each hand underneath each buttock, palm upward. Curl your fingertips upward, pressing through the buttocks until you feel a bony ridge against your fingertips. These are the sitting bones. Withdraw your hands. You should now be aware of the pressure of the sitting bones against the surface of the seat.

Slowly rock your pelvis back and forth until you find the upright position that allows neither a hollowed nor bulging lower back. See lllustration 43. This is the balancing point of the sitting bones.

If you do not use your sitting bones, two structural deviations occur. First, the pelvis tilts backward and drags the spine with it, eventually causing malformation and often pains in the lower back, and second, because the pelvis is not erect, the abdomen is forced to protrude.

The inner-margin ball of the foot is also important to balanced sitting.

To develop awareness of the inner-margin ball of the foot, slowly raise all your toes straight upward. Stretch and hold the toes raised a moment. Realize that when the toes are in the air, the forward part of each foot is pressing against the floor. This forward part is the ball of the foot.

Sense the pressure on the area of the ball of the foot that is in the back of

Illustration 44. The inner-margin ball of the foot.

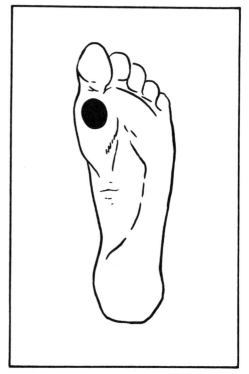

100

each big toe. It is this particular pressure point that is referred to as the inner-margin ball of the foot (See Illustration 44).

Now, slowly lower all the toes, being careful to lay them down straight, and continue to feel the inner-margin ball of the foot pressing against the floor.

From now on, when I say "ball of the foot" I shall be referring to the big-toe or inner-margin ball.

EXERCISE SCHEME 1: *The Balanced Sitting Position*

Sit toward the forward edge of a stool, or a firm, flat armless chair, squarely on the buttocks, as in Illustration 45.

Find the balancing point of the sitting bone.

Place both feet directly in front of you, parallel to each other, about two inches apart, as in Illustration 46. Make sure your legs are straight from heels to knees.

Press lightly onto the ball of each foot. Keep both knees and thighs

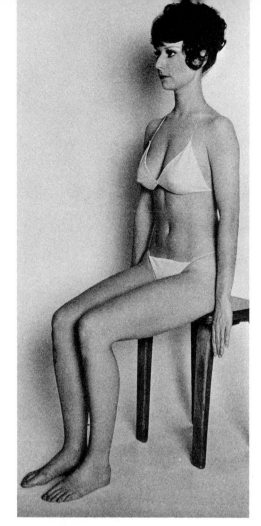

Illustration 45. The balanced sitting position.

Illustration 46. Correct parallel feet; *in*correct toe-out.

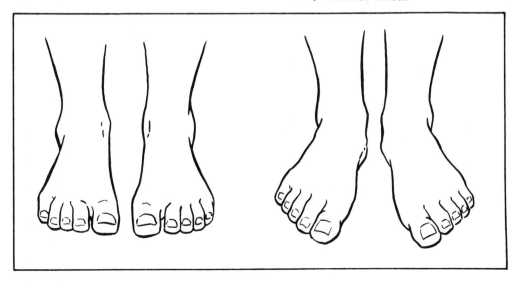

parallel to each other, about two inches apart.

With the two long back muscles, which are on either side of the spine, stretch the spine (including the neck) upward to an erect position. See Illustrations 47W and 48R, and observe the spine's normal S-curve. Look for the S-curve in your rear mirror.

Keep the shoulder tips down and, using the shoulder-blade muscles, draw both shoulder blades enough toward each other until they are flattened against the rib cage. Don't draw them together beyond flattening them, because you will then be in a distorted position.

Stretch both arms down at your sides, with the palms of the hands facing your body. Then rotate your arms inward in the shoulder sockets until your palms face the back.

This is the Balanced Sitting Position.

Slowly release all muscles used, from the top of your body downward.

This exercise will build the muscles necessary for correct and comfortable everyday sitting.

To Remember: The inner-margin ball of the foot (peroneus)—for ball pressure.

The long back muscles (sacrospinales) hold the spine erect.

Illustration 47. Skeletal view of sitting incorrectly.

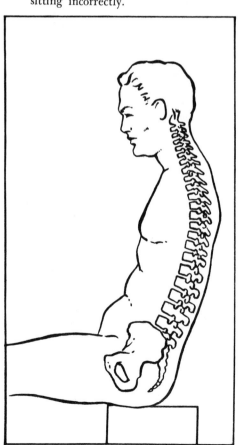

Illustration 48. Skeletal view of sitting correctly.

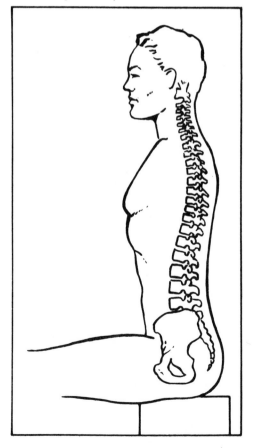

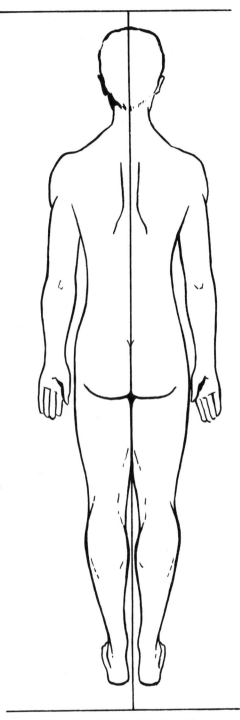

Illustration 49. The Median Plane.

The purpose of this exercise is to achieve a balanced distribution of the body weight and the correct alignment of the body masses. The exercise activates a range of muscles from the feet upward, notably those of the buttocks, the inner-margins of the thighs, the abdominal muscle, the long back muscles, the shoulder and neck muscles— all significant in shaping the body.

The position achieved here should always be used when beginning any subsequent exercises that are done while standing. It should not be used in the day's activities, however, because the tension of the muscles and the rigidity of the body are greater than needed when not formally exercising. But the Balanced Standing Position can provide a *model* for correct standing.

This exercise places a premium on *precision*. It begins with the feet, assuring that the bearing of body weight is accurate, and proceeds upward in sequence, identifying and activating muscles to perform their alignment functions correctly. (The exercise reaches the neck and head, and even extends to the position of the hands.)

It is important to note that the front and back of the body are actually divided into two symmetrical halves with a groove (middle line) running down the center of the trunk. In Illustration 49, the middle line is extended through the length of the body. The middle line is called the Median Plane.

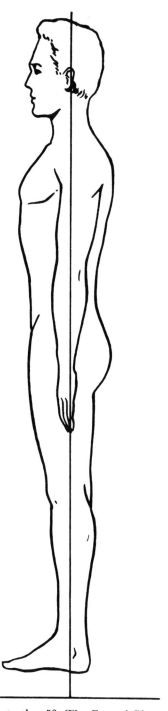

Illustration 50. The Frontal Plane.

The imaginary middle line for a figure in profile is called the Frontal Plane. (See Illustration 50.) When your body is correctly aligned, the Frontal Plane should run from the side of the crown, through the ear, shoulder tip, elbow, hip, knee and center of the foot.

EXERCISE SCHEME 2: *The Balanced Standing Position*

Stand unclothed between two full-length mirrors, as in Illustration 51.

The mirrors should be placed so that they give you a full front view and a three-quarter back view.

Illustration 51. The balanced standing position.

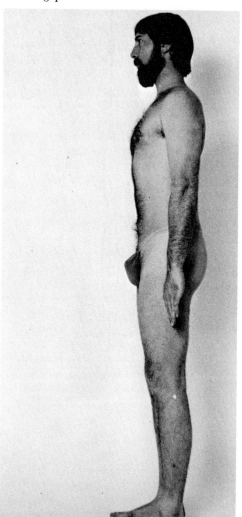

Through the front view you are able to judge the symmetry of the body, while the back view permits you to observe the important back muscles at work.

The two buttocks that make up the "seat" are muscles that can be contracted. Tactual aid can be used to help you identify them. Cup the hands over the buttocks and slowly tighten the buttock muscles, as shown in Illustration 52. Then slowly release the tension. You will feel the buttocks become firm and then soft again.

The muscles along the inner margin of the thighs are the adductors. They extend from the groin to the knee.

Illustration 52. Buttock muscle, tactual aid.

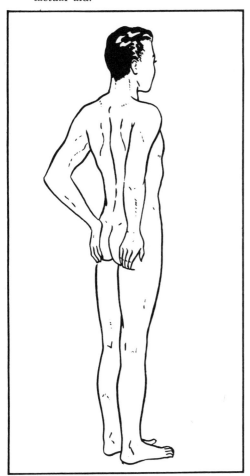

Place your feet about two inches apart and parallel to each other, with the toes of each foot on a line with the other.

Center your body weight over your insteps, halfway between the ball and heel of each foot.

Press downward slightly onto the ball of each foot, using pressure, *not body weight.* The ball pressure is meant to activate your arches and anchor your feet.

Starting from the center of your body, slowly tighten the adductor and buttock muscles and draw them toward each other. *Be sure not to shove these muscles together from the outer sides of your body.*

When you have tightened the adductors and buttocks, your knees should be relaxed, not pushed back and "locked," so that your legs are bent very slightly. Then to straighten your legs, pull up your kneecaps by using the muscles that run along the front of the thighs. These front thigh muscles are the quadriceps, and they extend from the knee to the groin area.

Starting at the base of your spine, draw your back upward by stretching the spine with the long back muscles which are on either side of the spinal column. The base of your spine is the lower back, the lumbar region. This stretching of the spine should be done as though you were drawing apart one vertebra from the other from the lumbar region upward.

Keeping the shoulder tips down, continue stretching the spine (including the vertebrae in back of the neck) so that you raise your head until your chin and the front of your neck form a right angle. Be aware that you are now using neck muscles to stretch apart seven spinal vertebrae in the back of your neck. This enables you to raise the crown of your head without a sense of straining the neck.

Now you have to square your shoulders and flatten your back. With the shoulder-blade muscles (rhomboideus) that are attached to your shoulder blades and your spine, draw your shoulder blades toward each other until they are flattened on either side of the spine. The upper-back muscles used here are the rhomboideus and trapezius, extending from each side of the spine. Sense how your shoulders are being straightened and observe in the back mirror the flattened shoulder blades and the heightened muscle definition of the trapezius.

Check to assure that the whole body is now erect and perpendicular. (Illustration 53W, shows an incorrect position, and Illustration 54R shows the correct position.)

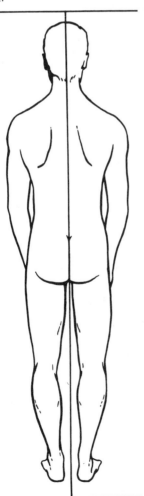

Illustration 53W. The median plane in the incorrect standing position.

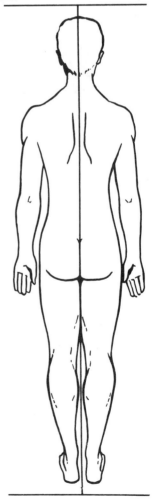

Illustration 54R. The median plane in the correct standing position.

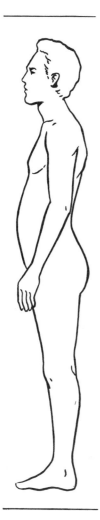

Illustration 55W. Side view of an incorrect standing position.

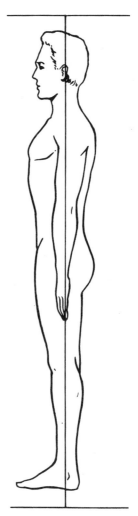

Illustration 56R. Side view of the correct standing position showing the frontal plane.

Now stand with your side to the mirror to determine whether you have achieved the correct position. Illustration 55W, of course, shows a wrong position. Illustration 56R again shows the Frontal Plane when the body is in the correct position.

To align the arms, begin by holding the shoulder blades flat as you stretch your arms downward from the shoulder tips to the fingertips, with the palms facing your thighs.

Now slowly rotate your arms inward in the shoulder socket, until your thumbs face the thighs and your palms face backward. This turning movement, so beneficial to the arms, begins at the shoulder joint, then reaches the elbow joint and ultimately the wrist joint. As you do it, be sure to keep your shoulder tips down and your shoulder blades flattened on either side of the spine.

Hold this position a few moments, then, in sequence, slowly relax all muscles used, from the head downward.

For normal standing, the position of the body should be basically the same as it is in the Balanced Standing Positions. Your hands, however, should hang naturally and comfortably at your sides. The muscles throughout the rest of your body should be less taut than in the exercise position, and your body should not be rigid. The Balanced Standing Position trains your body so that correct standing will become habitual.

To REMEMBER: The inner-margin ball of the foot (peroneus) "anchors" the feet and activates the arch.

The leg muscles, peroneus, adductors, quadriceps, hold the legs erect.

The pelvic muscles, buttocks, lower abdominals, hold the pelvis erect.

The long back muscles (sacrospinales) hold the trunk erect.

RHYTHMIC BREATHING

The purpose of this exercise scheme is to indicate the essentials of rhythmic breathing so that the breathing organs and the body processes can be sustained at maximum effectiveness. Furthermore, this exercise scheme works on muscles that many people do not know they have. We are all aware of our ribs, but what of their slender muscle strappings that guide rib movements in breathing? This exercise scheme disciplines and strengthens those muscles and establishes a beneficial breathing rhythm. The very pulsations of energy on which we depend for daily activity draw major sustenance from the oxygen we take in by this breathing rhythm.

The exercise movements call for rhythmical breathing in which the time required for inhalation exactly matches the time required for exhalation. In the process, the muscles are activated to spread the lower ribs apart and then bring them together again.

This spreading of the ribs can be felt tactually.

The anatomy of this exercise focuses on the main breathing muscles, the intercostals and the diaphragm. The intercostal muscles are between the ribs, lacing them together to form the chest cavity. The diaphragm is the partition which separates the abdomen from the rib cage.

Few of us are aware that these muscles can be exercised and that a full development of them can increase our breathing capacity and the flow of oxygen into the blood stream.

When these muscles are in tonic condition, they spread the ribs further apart and increase the capacity of the breathing organs to draw in air and oxygen.

But this alone is not enough. The capabilities for exhaling must also be expanded to the point of completely emptying the lungs and ridding the body of carbon dioxide. If we are short-breathed, it is usually not because we don't sufficiently breathe in, but because we forget to breathe out sufficiently.

Our anatomical arrangements are such that rhythmical deep breathing affects the contours of two areas. Most directly it improves the development of the chest.

In addition, the movements of the diaphragm will improve the outline of the upper abdominal area.

Illustration 57. Rhythmic breathing, tactual aid.

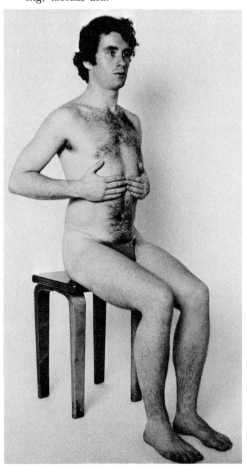

EXERCISE SCHEME 3:
Rhythmic Breathing

Take the Balanced Sitting Position.

Cup both hands over the lower ribs so that the fingertips touch as in Illustration 57.

Then gently press the hands against the lower ribs and inhale slowly, counting as you inhale and directing the rib cage response to the lower ribs, drawing them sideward and apart.

Avoid the usual breathing movement of drawing the rib cage upward until the upper ribs push the chest and breast outward.

As you breathe in, feel with your fingertips and the palms of your hands the muscles slowly drawing the ribs apart, spreading them sideways.

Recall the number of counts in inhaling. Open your mouth and breathe out audibly (making the sound of a sigh), timing your exhalation to match your inhalation. As you exhale direct your muscles to guide your ribs back to the middle line.

Repeat the exercise tactually several times.

Thereafter, do the exercise without cupping the hands over your lower ribs.

To Remember: The diaphragm and intercostals spread the ribs sideward and apart.

109

THE RHOMBOIDEUS—
SHOULDER-BLADE
MOVEMENTS

The purpose of these exercises is to strengthen and shape your back with special emphasis on the shoulder blades. The shoulder blades should lie flat against your rib cage and not poke out like wings.

The exercises also teach the correct way to raise and lower your arms, developing and shaping your arms and shoulders.

EXERCISE SCHEME 4:
The Rhomboideus, Sitting

Take the Balanced Sitting Position.

Increase the pressure slightly on your sitting bones.

Check to assure that your arms are straight down at your sides with palms facing *backward.*

Slowly bend both hands at the wrist joint until your fingertips point backward and the palms face upward.

While inhaling, use the muscles at the tops of your arms (front deltoids) to slowly raise both arms forward and upward until they are overhead. Keep your hands relaxed. Your arms should be straight and parallel to each other.

When your arms are overhead, exhale as you now slowly point your fingers to the ceiling, moving your hands from the wrists. See Illustration 58.

Inhale as you now slowly slant your hands sideways.

Exhale, and by using your shoulder-blade muscles to draw the shoulder

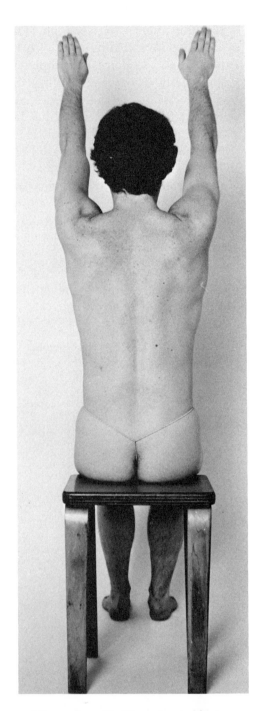

Illustration 58. The rhomboideus arm movement.

110

blades toward each other, slowly lower your arms straight sideward. See Illustrations 59 and 60.

When your arms are straight down, point your fingers to the floor. Rotate your arms inward in the shoulder socket until the palms face the back, returning to the Balanced Sitting Position.

Now slowly release all muscle tension from the top of your neck downward.

To Remember: The muscle which raises the arm forward and upward is located at the top of the arm and is called the front deltoid.

The lowering of the arm sideward involves three back muscles, the rhomboideus, the trapezius, and the latissimus dorsi.

The rhomboideus (see Illustrations 61 and 62) and trapezius draw the shoulder blades toward each other and

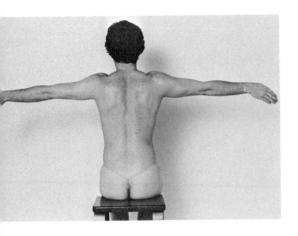

Illustrations 59 and 60. The rhomboideus arm movement.

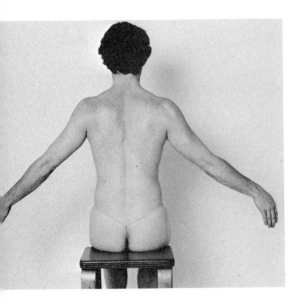

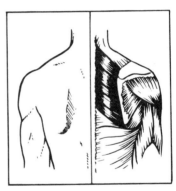

Illustration 61. The rhomboideus muscle of the back, relaxed.

Illustration 62. The rhomboideus muscle of the back, contracted.

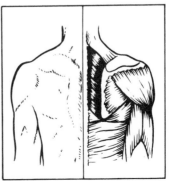

lower the arms to a little below shoulder height. After that, the muscle known as the "corset of the body" (latissimus dorsi) takes over the job of lowering the arm, and when it is in good condition it keeps the waistline trim.

EXERCISE SCHEME 5: *The Rhomboideus, Standing*

Take the Balanced Standing Position.

Increase the pressure slightly on the inner-margin ball of each foot.

Make sure that your body is erect, your buttock and adductor muscles are tight, your legs are straight with kneecaps pulled up, your shoulder tips are down, and your arms stretched down at your sides with the palms facing back.

Slowly bend your hands back at the wrist.

Inhale and, using your deltoids at the top of your arms, slowly raise your arms forward and upward until they are overhead, keeping your hands relaxed. Then exhale and use your wrists to turn your hands up so that your fingers point to the ceiling.

Be sure to keep your arms straight and parallel to each other and your shoulder tips down.

Now inhale and slowly slant your hands sideways from the wrist joint until your fingertips point to the side. This prepares you to lower your arms by means of the shoulder-blade muscles, as in Illustration 63.

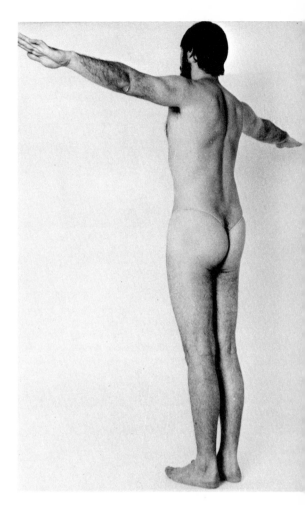

Illustration 63. The rhomboideus movement, standing.

Exhale and, by drawing the shoulder blades toward each other, slowly lower your arms sideward until the hands touch your thighs. Then point your fingers to the floor.

Rotate your arms inward in the shoulder sockets until the palms face the back.

You have now returned to the Balanced Standing Position.

112

Slowly release muscle tension from the top downward.

To Remember: The front deltoid raises the arms forward and upward.

The rhomboideus, trapezius, and latissimus dorsi lower the arms sideward.

THE PELVIC ROCK

The aim of this exercise is to make you aware of and to teach you to control one of the most important parts of the body, the pelvis.

The spine is attached to the pelvis, and it depends on the pelvis to provide it with the foundation it needs. In order for the spine to have a firm, solid foundation, the pelvis must be in an erect position.

In the sitting position, an erect pelvis can only be maintained by sitting on the balancing point of the sitting bones.

If the sitting bones are not used in sitting, the pelvis tilts back and the spine cannot maintain its normal S-curve. This causes the trunk to slump and the abdomen to bulge.

EXERCISE SCHEME 6: *The Pelvic Rock, Sitting*

Take the Balanced Sitting Position.

Inhale as you slowly tilt your pelvis forward, hollowing the back.

Move only your pelvis, not your trunk.

Hold this position for a moment and then exhale as you allow the pelvis to slowly fall back, beyond the Balanced Sitting Position, until your lower back slightly bulges outward. No muscles are required for this movement—giving in to gravity will make your pelvis fall back by itself. See Illustration 64.

Repeat this pelvic rocking exercise slowly several times.

Return to the Balanced Sitting Position before releasing all muscles used from the top downward.

Illustration 64. The pelvic rock, sitting, showing the pelvis tilted forward, then falling back into a straight position, and finally tilted back.

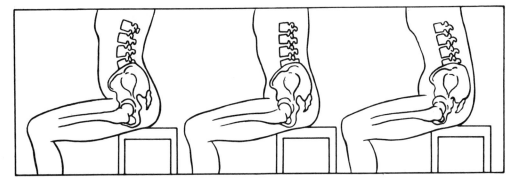

To Remember: The long back muscles tilt the pelvis forward.

THE PELVIC ROCK, STANDING

The purpose of this exercise is to increase the movability of the lower spine, and to improve the quality of the buttock muscles and the lower section of the abdomen. It draws attention to the relation between the pelvic position and the spine, emphasizing the normal erect position of the pelvis and the normal S-curve of the lower spine. It also increases blood circulation in the lower abdominal cavity.

This is a very effective movement for incipient hernia and constitutes the remedial exercise for a lordotic condition of the lumbar region (sway back).

It is not advisable to use this movement when the lumbar region of the spine is normal or over-flexible.

The pelvic-rocking movement should not be used during pregnancy.

Exercise Scheme 7: *The Pelvic Rock, Standing*

Take the Balanced Standing Position.

Inhale.

As you begin to exhale, slowly draw your buttocks together, then under and simultaneously draw the lowest part of your abdomen in and up. See Illustration 65. You will note that this is a very slight movement, but you are nonetheless rocking your

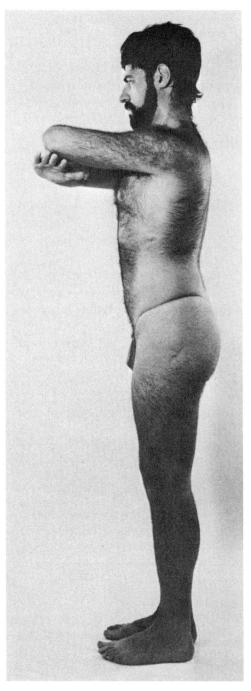

Illustration 65. The pelvic rock forward.

114

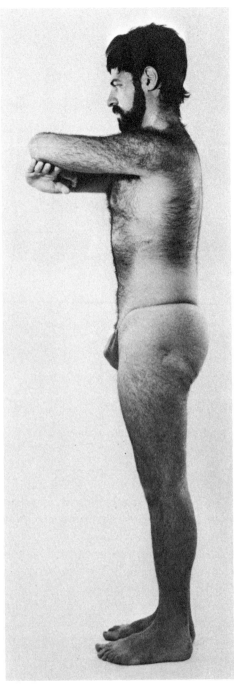

Illustration 66. The pelvic rock back until it is erect.

pelvis down in back and correspondingly up in front.

Now inhale as you slowly release the tension of your buttock and abdominal muscles while simultaneously using the lowest part of the long back muscles to raise the back of your pelvis (sacrum). In this way you rock your pelvis down in front, as in Illustration 66.

Now exhale while again slowly drawing your buttocks tightly together, then under, and your lower abdomen in and up—but only until your pelvis is held erect with the lumbar region of your spine assuming its normal S-curve. Thus, you have returned to the Balanced Standing Position by partially rocking your pelvis —downward in back and correspondingly upward at the pubic bone in front.

TO REMEMBER: The buttock muscles and lower abdominal muscles lower the sacrum and raise the pubic bone.

The lower section of the long back muscles raises the sacrum.

FORWARD TRUNK BENDING

The purpose of this exercise is to increase the flexibility of the spine —especially the lumbar area.

This exercise also considerably improves the quality of the abdominal area. It reduces the accumulation of fat over the abdominal muscles, and it is particularly helpful in improving

115

the weakness known as prolapsed inner organs.

Since nearly all of our movements
are in a forward direction and require
bending, to a lesser or greater degree,
the Round Forward Trunk Bend exercise is the most important of all the
exercises.

If after learning the Round Forward Trunk Bend you apply its principles to all bending movements, the
reward will be great—a trimmer,
flatter, stronger abdomen and a much
stronger lumbar region that should be
free from aches and pains.

EXERCISE SCHEME 8: *The Round
Forward Trunk Bend*

Take the Balanced Standing Position.

Press down onto the ball of each
foot. Bend your hands back at the
wrists, inhale, and use the front deltoids to raise your arms forward and
upward until they are overhead. Then
exhale as you point your fingers to the
ceiling.

Inhale as you bend the hands back.

Now exhale as you slowly begin to
draw your tightened buttocks carefully under. Simultaneously draw in
and up the lowest section of the abdominal muscle, allowing the abdominal muscle to begin drawing the trunk
forward from its lowest section (lumbar region).

Be careful to continue holding your
arms at the ears, and to press firmly
onto the ball of each foot.

Continue to draw your abdomen in
and up and to draw your buttocks

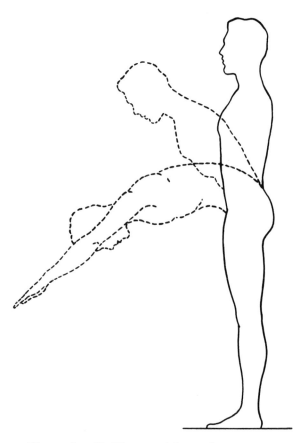

Illustration 67. The round forward
trunk bend.

under, thus bending the spine forward and downward until you have
bent the entire spine in an arc. Note
Illustration 67.

Now you are prepared to raise your
back with the long back muscles.

Bend your hands down.

Again, press firmly onto the ball of
each foot and draw your buttocks under. Now inhale and, starting at the
lowest section of your long back muscles, slowly begin to raise the entire
trunk, as in Illustration 68. Continue
to raise your trunk with the long back

116

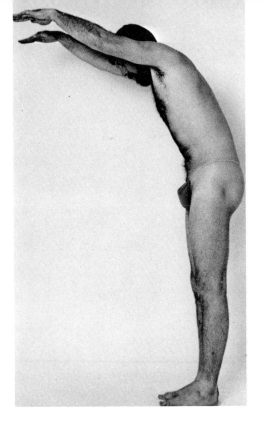

Illustration 68. Using the long back muscles to raise the trunk.

muscles, section after section, until the entire spine is held erect and your arms are overhead.

Then exhale as you use your wrists to point your fingers to the ceiling.

Inhale as you slant your hands sideward, and exhale as you use the shoulder-blade muscles to slowly lower your arms straight sideward.

Point your fingers to the floor and rotate your arms inward until the palms face the back, returning to the Balanced Standing Position.

Release all muscle contractions from the top downward.

To Remember: The abdominal muscle (rectus abdominis) bends the trunk forward.

The long back muscles (sacrospinales) raise the trunk.

All leg muscles keep the legs as erect as possible.

The buttock muscles (gluteus maximus) hold the pelvis erect.

SIDE TRUNK BENDING

The purpose of this exercise is to improve the flexibility of the spine in a sideward direction. This exercise will also slenderize the waistline and the abdominal area.

Exercise Scheme 9A: *The Side Trunk, Sitting*

Take the Balanced Sitting Position. Increase the pressure slightly on your sitting bones.

Illustration 69. The side trunk bend.

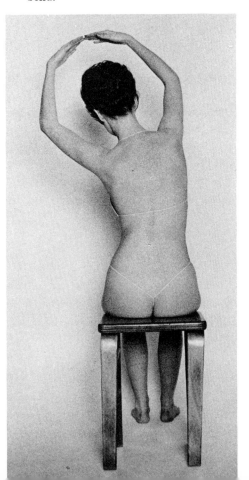

Rotate both arms outward in the shoulder sockets. Inhale, and use the upper part of your arms (middle deltoid) to raise them sideward (palms up) until they are overhead (palms facing each other). Allow your fingertips to touch. Exhale, and as you lower your shoulder tips keep your fingertips touching.

Inhale, and starting on your right side at your waistline, slowly stretch the right side of your trunk upward, poking your ribs out to the right and leaning your trunk over to the left, as in Illustration 69.

Hold this position as you exhale.

Inhale as, from your waist, you slowly move your trunk back to an erect position. Hold this position as you exhale.

Then inhale, and starting on your left side at your waistline, slowly stretch upward, poking your ribs out to the left and leaning over to the right. Hold this position as you exhale.

Now inhale, and slowly move your trunk back to an erect position.

Exhale, and with the shoulder blade muscles, lower your arms sideward, keeping the arms rotated out until your hands reach your thighs.

Rotate your arms inward until the palms face the back, returning to the Balanced Sitting Position.

Release all muscle tension from the top downward.

To Remember: The long back muscles (sacrospinales) bend the spine to the side.

The muscles between the ribs (in-tercostals) poke out the ribs and spread them apart.

THE SIDE TRUNK BEND, STANDING

The purpose of this exercise is to improve the flexibility of the spine as well as to slenderize and shape the waistline and abdomen.

Exercise Scheme 9B: *The Side Trunk Bend, Standing*

Take the Balanced Standing Position.

Rotate both arms outward and raise them sideward overhead until the palms face each other and the fingertips touch.

Press firmly onto the ball of each foot and make sure that your buttocks and adductors are tight and that the lower abdomen is drawn in and up.

As you do the following bending movements, be very careful to hold your weight evenly over both legs and to keep your arms at the sides of your ears.

Now slowly breathe in and simultaneously begin to draw the left side of your ribs gradually outward and upward. Continue to gradually spread your ribs and at the same time stretch the entire spine until you have bent your trunk over to your right side—but without making a kink over your right waistline.

Hold this position while exhaling.

Be certain to continue holding your weight evenly over both legs and to keep your arms at the side of your ears.

Now press again onto the ball of each foot and draw your buttocks and adductors tightly together.

Inhale, and using the long back muscles, begin at your left waistline to draw your trunk slowly upward. Continue to stretch and to raise your trunk while simultaneously lowering your left ribs, starting from the bottom and working upward, until your entire spine has been erected again.

Exhale while using the shoulder-blade muscles to lower your arms sideward.

Repeat the exercise, but this time use the right as the active side and bend your trunk to the left.

Release all muscles used from the top downward.

TO REMEMBER: The long back muscles (sacrospinales) bend the spine sideward.

The muscles between the ribs (intercostals) poke out the ribs and spread them sideward.

THE BREAST MUSCLE

The purpose of this exercise is to build the chest, to lift and firm the breasts, and to help you sit and stand in an erect position.

EXERCISE SCHEME 10A: *The Breast Muscle Exercise, Sitting*

Take the Balanced Sitting Position. Increase the pressure slightly on the sitting bones.

As a tactual aid, begin by using the middle deltoid to raise your left arm sideward to shoulder height. Cup your right hand over the left breast muscle (pectoralis) as in Illustration 70. As you slowly move your *left* arm toward the center of the body, you will feel the thickening of the breast muscle on the left side.

It is important that you keep your left arm relaxed and passive so that the movement of your arm can originate at the breast muscle.

Continue moving your arm forward until it passes the center of the body. Then, using the *shoulder-blade muscles*, move your left arm back to your side, keeping your arm at shoulder height. Continuing to use the shoul-

Illustration 70. The breast muscle, tactual aid.

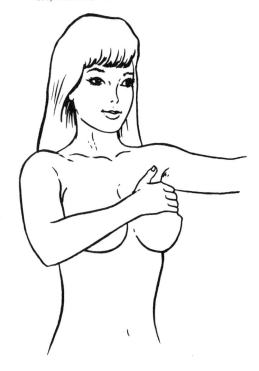

der-blade muscles, slowly lower your arm sideward.

Repeat the use of tactual aid with your right arm.

After this, inhale as you use the middle deltoids to raise both arms sideward to above shoulder height (see Illustration 71), and while ex-

Illustration 71. The breast muscle exercise, sitting.

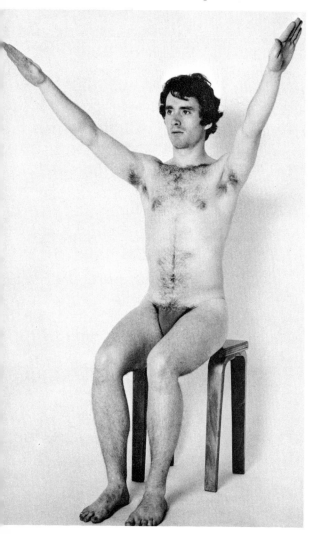

haling, use the breast muscle to move both your arms slowly toward the middle line until your hands cross each other in front.

Now inhale as you use the shoulder-blade muscles to move both arms slowly back to your sides at shoulder level.

Exhale, and continuing to use the shoulder-blade muscles, slowly lower your arms sideward.

Rotate your arms inward until the palms face the back, returning to the Balanced Sitting Position before releasing all tension from the top downward.

You will benefit greatly by also doing this exercise with your arms raised to only shoulder height. I usually suggest to my students that they first learn to do the exercise with their arms raised to a diagonal position above shoulder height. When doing the exercise four times daily thereafter, they alternate the height of their arms—the first time with their arms raised to above shoulder height, the second time with their arms raised to just shoulder height, and so on. If you follow this procedure you will exercise different parts of the breast muscle and further improve its condition.

To REMEMBER: Muscles at the top of the arms (middle deltoids) raise the arm sideward.

The breast muscle (pectoralis) draws the arms from the side toward the middle line.

The shoulder-blade muscles (middle and lower trapezius) draw the shoulder blades toward the middle line.

The "corset of the body" (latissimus) lowers the arms from shoulder height.

EXERCISE SCHEME 10B: *The Breast Muscle Exercise, Standing*

Take the Balanced Standing Position.

Increase the pressure onto the ball of the foot and be sure that your buttock and adductor muscles are tight.

Inhale and use the middle deltoids to raise your arms sideward to above shoulder height, as in Illustration 72.

Exhale, and use the breast muscle to slowly draw your arms forward. Your shoulder blades will simultaneously glide apart.

Keep your arms as passive as possible, and you will sense the contraction of the breast muscle.

Continue to draw your arms forward until your wrists cross in front of you.

Now inhale and use your shoulder-blade muscles to slowly draw your shoulder blades toward each other and spread your arms sideward.

Be sure to keep your arms shoulder height and as passive as possible.

When your arms have reached the side, exhale and slowly lower them sideward.

Rotate your arms inward, as usual, and release all muscle contractions from the top downward.

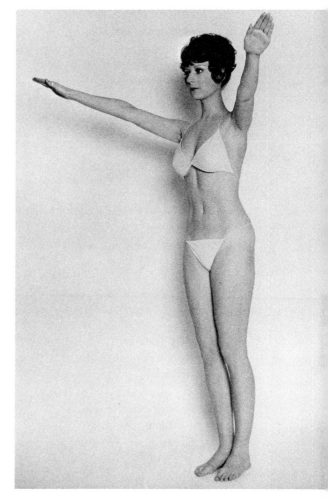

Illustration 72. The breast muscle exercise, standing.

After you have learned how to do this exercise correctly, it, too, should be done with your arms alternately above shoulder height and at shoulder height.

TO REMEMBER: The breast muscle (pectoralis) draws the arms from the side toward the center of the body.

121

The shoulder-blade muscles (middle and lower trapezius) draw the arms from the center of the body to the side.

The "corset of the body" (latissimus) lowers the arm sideward from shoulder height.

NECK AND CHIN LINE

The purpose of this exercise is to slenderize and shape the neck and to prevent or eliminate a double chin.

EXERCISE SCHEME 11A: *The Round Forward Neck Bend, Seated*

Take the Balanced Sitting Position.
Increase the pressure slightly on the sitting bones.

Beginning at the lower back, use the long back muscles to stretch the spine and draw your trunk upward as tall as possible. Remember to stretch the spine as though the vertebrae were being slightly separated from each other. Continue the stretch up through the seven vertebrae of the back of the neck.

Slowly raise your chin and move it slightly forward so that it forms a right angle with the front of the neck.

Check the back mirror to assure that your shoulder tips are down and your shoulder blades are flat against your rib cage.

Your arms should hang relaxed at your sides.

Inhale.

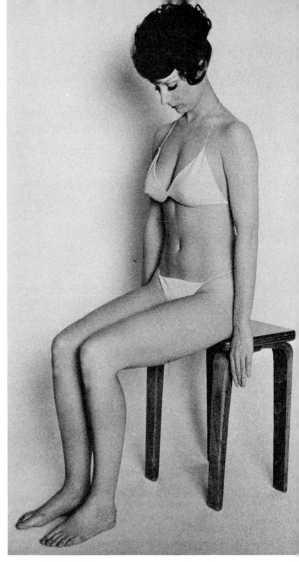

Illustration 73. Neck bend, forward.

Now exhale while from the base of the back of your neck you slowly bend the neck forward, as though you were rounding the back of your neck and pushing your head forward. Your neck should form an arc as your chin moves downward, as in Illustration 73.

Continue the movement until the

122

entire back of your neck is curved forward.

Avoid tilting your head to one side.

Hold your head in this position for several seconds: neck forming a curve, head bent as though the forehead is being pushed forward, chin down and forming an arc of the neck.

Now, on an inhalation, slowly reverse the direction of movement by raising your head and straightening your neck. Move your head and neck with the muscles that are in back of the neck as though, beginning at the bottom, you were returning the seven vertebrae successively into position.

Continue this movement until your entire neck column is erect and your head is straight, with your chin forward and forming a right angle with your neck.

Exhale and hold this straightened position several seconds.

Relax your body by releasing the muscles from the top downward.

Do this movement three times. Rest for a minute before continuing with the Side Neck Bend.

To Remember: The back of the neck muscles (cervical section of the sacrospinales) erect the neck column.

NECK AND CHIN LINE

This exercise reinforces the Round Forward Neck Bend. It increases flexibility of the neck and helps to hold the head erect and straight.

Exercise Scheme 11B: *The Side Neck Bend, Sitting*

Take the Balanced Sitting Position.

Inhale, and use the back neck muscles to stretch the muscles on the *right* side of your neck while slowly bending your head straight to the *left*.

Continue to hold your shoulder tips down and your shoulder blades together and flat.

Make sure that your head does not lean forward and that the position of your chin is maintained in a right angle with your neck.

Now exhale as you slowly straighten your neck and raise your head until upright. Use the muscles *back of the neck* to slowly raise your head; as you do this, you should use the *left* neck muscles to offer some resistance—as though your head itself were resisting being straightened—but avoid any sense of strain.

Hold your head upright and straight for a moment or two.

Then repeat this movement on the other side, beginning by using the back of the neck muscles to stretch the muscles on the *left* side of your neck.

Do this sideward neck bending three times on each side before returning to the Balanced Sitting Position.

Having returned to the Balanced Sitting Position, remain this way several seconds and then slowly relax the muscles of the body from the head downward.

To Remember: The back of the

neck muscles (cervical section of the sacrospinales) erect the neck column.

NOTE: After this movement scheme has been learned, you may do the movements standing, being certain, however, to maintain the Balanced Standing Position throughout.

FOOT EXERCISES

The purpose of the toe movement exercise is to develop the stretcher muscles of the toes, and to improve the shape and increase the strength of the foot.

By achieving a functionally sound use of the foot, crooked toes can be straightened and bunions eliminated.

This exercise also helps you to become aware of and locate the ball of the foot.

The exercise seems simple enough: It is merely a raising and stretching apart of the toes. Yet most people find it difficult at first, for clawing the toes into the ground is commonplace but to raise them up is unusual. Patiently and gradually, however, the natural movement of toe raising can be renewed.

EXERCISE SCHEME 12A: *Toe Raising*

Take the Balanced Sitting Position.
Using the muscles on the margin of your instep, slowly raise your toes while inhaling in the manner you learned in Exercise 2.

Strive to raise all toes simultaneously, moving them together to the same height. Raise them as high as you can

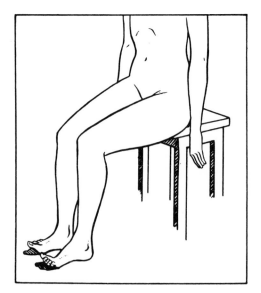

Illustration 74. Toes raised.

with the goal of pointing them straight upward, as in Illustration 74.

Initially be content with raising your toes slightly, but gradually raise them higher and higher as the stretcher muscles of the toes strengthen.

Hold your toes raised for several seconds as you exhale.

Note what this movement involves. The heel and the ball of the feet remain solidly on the ground. Foot muscles have been activated which raise the middle of the foot, heightening the arch.

Now inhale.

Exhale as you lower your toes slowly, straightening them and stretching them apart as you do so. Then gently lay your toes down on the ground.

Slowly release all muscles in sequence, starting from the top, downward.

To Remember: The stretcher muscles of the toes are situated on the instep of the foot.

FOOT EXERCISES (CONTINUED)

In the sitting position, the purpose of the heel raising and lowering is different from the standing position, because in the standing position the body weight is distributed differently.

In the seated position the flexibility of all joints of the foot, with the exception of the toes, is improved. The position of all middle foot bones, especially those of the instep, is improved.

Raising and lowering of the heels while in the sitting position also improves the condition of the calf muscle. It brings improved circulation to all parts of the foot, ankle-joint, and lower leg.

It also teaches the proper use of the calf muscle. That knowledge can then be applied to the many daily motions in which heel raising is necessary, such as walking, going up or downstairs, and so on.

Finally, it points out the need for the use of the big-toe ball whenever the heel-raising and lowering motion is performed.

EXERCISE SCHEME 12B: *Heel Raising, Sitting*

Take the Balanced Sitting Position.
Slowly increase the pressure on the ball of each foot.

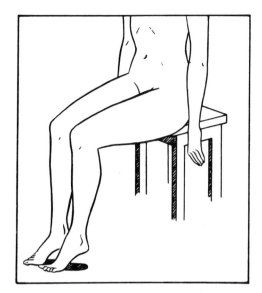

Illustration 75. Heels raised.

Inhale and with your calf muscles slowly begin to raise your heels. Try to raise your heels on a straight line, keeping them parallel to each other, as in Illustration 75. Without releasing the ball of the foot pressure, continue raising your heels until they have been fully elevated.

Keep your knees the same distance apart as your feet.

Exhale as you slowly release the tension of the calf muscles and simultaneously lower your heels, keeping them parallel to each other and still retaining the ball of the foot pressure.

Slowly release all muscles in sequence, starting from the top.

To Remember: The calf muscles (triceps surae) raise the heels.

The inner-margin ball of the foot (peroneus) keeps the foot in place.

HEEL RAISING

The purpose of this exercise is to learn to balance yourself on the ball of the foot by using the balancing muscles, the adductors.

This exercise also develops and shapes the calf and slenderizes the ankle joint.

EXERCISE SCHEME 12C: *Heel Raising, Standing*

Take the Balanced Standing Position.

Increase the pressure on the ball of each foot.

As you begin to inhale use your calf muscles to slowly raise your heels off the ground, shifting the leg weight to the ball of the foot. The weight should be shifted along the inner margin of the instep.

Be sure to move slowly until the weight has been shifted to the ball of the foot and to stop there, without extending the movement to the toes.

Now exhale as you slowly release your calf muscles and lower your heels to the ground.

Keep the pressure on the ball of each foot until your heels touch the ground.

Release the muscle contractions from the head downward.

TO REMEMBER: The calf muscles (triceps surae) raise the heels.

The inner-margin ball of the foot (peroneus) holds the weight on the ball of the foot.

126

THE SQUAT

The purpose of this exercise is to increase the flexibility of the knee joints, to improve the shape of the thighs, and to teach correct body balance. It also improves the condition of all leg and foot joints.

EXERCISE SCHEME 13: *The Squat*

Take the Balanced Standing Position.

Bend your hands back at the wrists.

Inhale as you raise your arms forward and upward until they are overhead.

Exhale as you point your fingers to the ceiling.

Illustration 76. The squat.

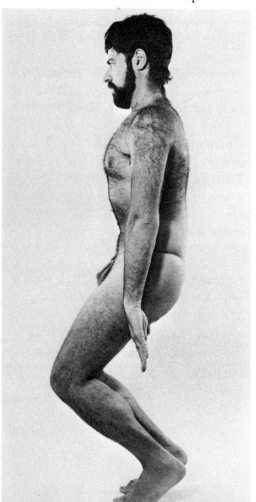

Increase the pressure on the ball of each foot and be sure that your buttocks and adductors are tight.

Inhale as you use your calf muscles to slowly raise your heels.

Now exhale as you *slowly* shove the knees forward by tucking under your tightened buttocks. See Illustration 76.

The extent of downward leg movement should match the tension of the buttock muscles. Stop the movement when the tension of the buttocks is about to release.

Keep your knees parallel to each other and your back stretched and straight.

Now inhale as you again slightly tuck under your tightened buttocks, and begin to stretch your knees, continuing to do so until your knees are straight and stretched.

Now exhale as, releasing your calf muscles, you slowly lower your heels.

Be sure to keep your feet parallel to each other during the raising and lowering of your heels.

Now inhale as you slant your hands sideward, and exhale as you use your shoulder-blade muscles to lower your arms straight sideward.

Point your fingers to the floor; rotate your arms inward until the palms face the back, returning to the Balanced Standing Position before releasing tension of all the muscles used.

To REMEMBER: The calf muscles (triceps surae) raise the heels.

The inner-margin ball of the foot (peroneus) holds the body weight forward.

WALKING

The main purpose of this exercise is to teach functional walking. However, there are additional benefits. The legs and feet are strengthened and shaped, the ankle joints are slenderized. The exercise also has a beneficial effect on flat feet.

EXERCISE SCHEME 14: *The Stiff-Legged Walk, Forward*

Take the Balanced Standing Position. Allow your arms to hang free at your sides.

Keeping the muscles of your pelvis tight, use the calf muscles to slowly raise your heels.

Illustration 77. The stiff-legged walk.

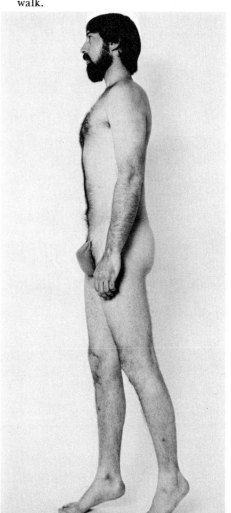

Begin to take short, quick, even steps straight forward, moving from the top of the leg. See Illustration 77.

Keep your knees and ankles stiff.

At first take only a few steps forward, being sure to maintain the Balanced Standing Position. As you become familiar with the exercise and find it easier to do, increase the number of steps you take.

When you want to stop, bring your feet together and release the calf muscles to slowly lower your heels.

This exercise can be done backward and sideward also, but be sure to do each movement separately. Do not combine forward walking with backward or sideward walking.

When you have learned these exercises they can be done at any time without removing your clothes. Remove only your shoes and be sure to walk on a firm, flat, resilient surface, such as a rug or grass.

To Remember: The calf muscles (triceps surae) raise the heels and lock the ankle joints.

The inner-margin ball of the foot (peroneus) and inner thigh muscles (adductors) keep the transfer of the body weight close to the Median Plane.

The front thigh muscles (quadriceps) keep the knees extended.

The buttock muscle (glutaeus maximus) on that side which carries the body weight balances the pelvis.

The long back muscles (sacrospinales) balance and hold the spine erect.

The shoulder-blade muscles (trapezius) hold the upper back erect and control the arm position.